101

Body-Sculpting
Workouts &
Nutrition Plans

FOR WOMEN

ACKNOWLEDGEMENTS

This publication is based on articles written by Karen Ansel, MS, RD, David Barr, CSCS, CISSN, Jordana Brown, Jon Finkel, Rob Fitzgerald, Anna Lee, Brad McCray, Jimmy Peña, MS, CSCS, Jim Stoppani, PhD, Mark Thorpe, Eric Velazquez, Roy M. Wallack, Kelly Wangard, Joe Wuebben

Cover photography by Marc Royce

Photography and illustrations by Alicia Buelow, Michael Darter, David Faught, Naj Jamai, John Kelly, Ian Logan, Rick Lohre, Karen Maze, Mike Medby, Pornchai Mittongtare, Marc Royce, Cory Sorensen

Project editor is Mark Thorpe

Project managing editor is Kristina Haar

Project copy editor is Jenny Gardner

Project creative director is Michael Touna

Project design assistant is Brandi Centeno

Photo assistant is Arlene Silver

Founding chairman is Joe Weider. Chairman and CEO of American Media, Inc., is David Pecker

This book is available in quantity at special discounts for your group or organization. For further information, contact:

Triumph Books
542 S. Dearborn St., Ste. 750
Chicago, IL 60605
(312) 939-3330
fax (312) 663-3557
www.triumphbooks.com

ISBN: 978-1-60078-514-6

Printed in U.S.A.

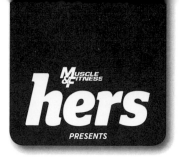

101
Body-Sculpting
Workouts &
Nutrition Plans

FOR WOMEN

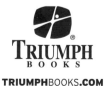

TRIUMPH
BOOKS

TRIUMPHBOOKS**.COM**

Contents

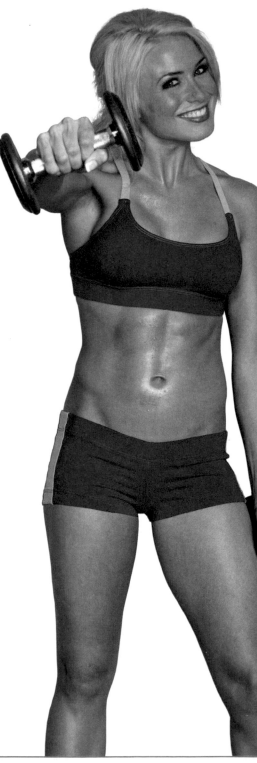

MARC ROYCE

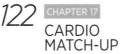
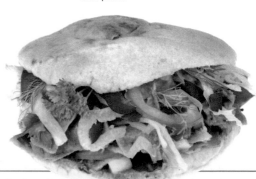

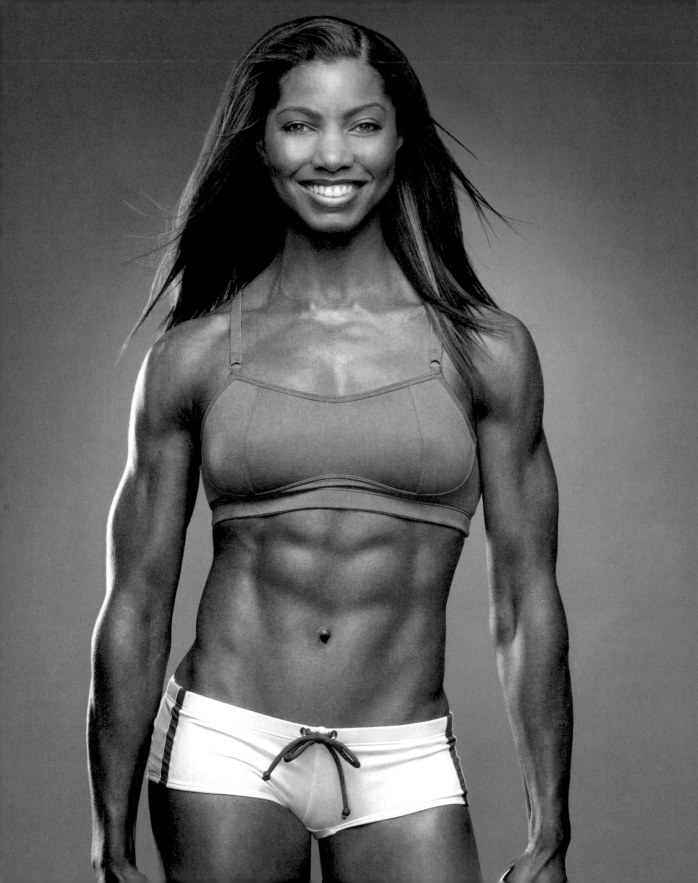

Chapter 1

Split Decision

Deciding which bodyparts to train together can be a real puzzle. We solve it for you

Chapter 1

To make noticeable improvements in your physique over weeks and months, you need to know how to change up your training. Whether through variables such as exercise and weight selection, sets and reps, or even your rest periods between sets, continually tweaking your workouts helps stave off plateaus and keeps the beneficial muscular adaptations coming. But before you can even consider altering your training variables, you need to decide on your training split. The split you use determines how frequently you work out each week, how often you exercise each muscle group in a week and what bodyparts get trained together.

Your current split may be something you adopted from a training partner or lifted from a popular fitness competitor's split presented in M&F HERS. While it might be good, it may not be the best split for you. And even if it's a great split, you should change it up from time to time as you do other training variables to prompt the gains you're looking for.

Why? For one thing, if you keep your training split the same month after month, your muscles will adapt and stagnate, limiting your progress. Two, if you train the same bodyparts in the same order every time, the muscles you hit later in the routine can't be worked with the same intensity as the ones trained first, again limiting your results.

While an endless combination of training splits exist, several fit a variety of experience levels and schedules. Here we lay out the four most common splits, and in "Trial Separation" at the end of this chapter we provide a way to try them all over the course of 12 weeks to help you gauge which ones work better for you.

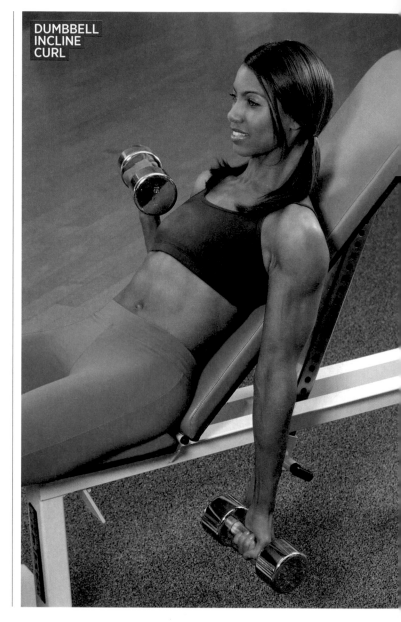

DUMBBELL INCLINE CURL

SPLIT NO. 1

Whole-Body

Three Days Per Week

Here you simply train the entire body each time you go to the gym. Typically, most whole-body workouts use only 1–2 exercises per muscle group with total sets per bodypart rarely exceeding six. This allows you to train each bodypart more frequently because it receives a limited amount of stress in each workout. The less stress a muscle receives, the faster it can recover and be trained again.

Although typically considered a beginner split, the whole-body option can also work well for advanced lifters. Training such a large number of muscle groups in each workout boosts growth-hormone levels, which helps to encourage muscle growth as well as fat-burning. Whole-body training also activates a greater amount of enzymes in muscles that turn on fat-burning processes.

In addition, research from St. Francis Xavier University (Antigonish, Nova Scotia, Canada) shows that female and male subjects who trained each muscle group three times per week had upper-body strength gains 8% greater and muscle mass gains 300% greater than those who trained twice a week. This was despite the fact that each group completed the same number of sets per bodypart, which means the three-times-per-week trainees did fewer sets per workout. So if you currently train each muscle group once a week for about 12 sets each, training each with four sets three times a week on a whole-body split instead will allow you to do the same number of sets per week but may enhance your results.

The simplest way to use the whole-body approach is to train on Monday, Wednesday and Friday, thus allowing at least one full day of rest between workouts. Of course, any three days that provide at least one day of rest between workouts will do, such as a Tuesday, Thursday and Saturday schedule. Be sure to do a different exercise for every muscle group in each of the three workouts per week to avoid staleness, and alternate the order of the bodyparts you train, being sure to move weak muscle groups earlier in the workout on some days. Our sample program accomplishes both of these goals to optimize your results.

MONDAY

BODYPART	EXERCISE	SETS/REPS
Chest	Dumbbell Incline Flye	4/10–12
Shoulders	Upright Row	4/10–12
Triceps	Pushdown	4/10–12
Quads	Leg Extension	3/10–12
Back	Lat Pulldown	4/10–12
Biceps	Dumbbell Incline Curl	4/10–12
Hamstrings	Lying Leg Curl	3/10–12
Abs	Reverse Crunch	4/12–15
Calves	Standing Calf Raise	4/10–12

WEDNESDAY

BODYPART	EXERCISE	SETS/REPS
Quads/Hams/Glutes	Squat	4/6–8
Chest	Dumbbell Bench Press	4/6–8
Back	Seated Cable Row	4/6–8
Shoulders	Dumbbell Overhead Press	4/6–8
Biceps	Barbell Curl	4/6–8
Triceps	Lying Triceps Extension	4/6–8
Calves	Seated Calf Raise	4/12–15
Abs	Hanging Leg Raise	4/10–12

FRIDAY

BODYPART	EXERCISE	SETS/REPS
Back	Barbell Row	4/15–20
Biceps	Preacher Curl	4/15–20
Quads/Hams/Glutes	Dumbbell Lunge	4/15–20
Calves	Leg-Press Calf Raise	4/15–20
Chest	Cable Crossover	4/15–20
Shoulders	Lateral Raise	4/15–20
Triceps	Overhead Triceps Extension	4/15–20
Abs	Crunch	4/15–20

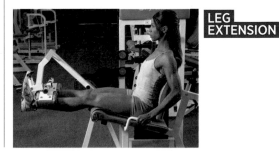

LEG EXTENSION

SPLIT NO. 2
Upper/Lower-Body
Four Days Per Week

In this split you break the body into upper (chest, back, shoulders, biceps and triceps) and lower (quads, hams, calves, glutes and abs) muscle groups. You can train each bodypart twice per week, in two upper-body and two lower-body workouts.

Because you split the entire body into two sessions, you can do more sets for each muscle group than in the whole-body split. It also allows you to train with a little more intensity, since you have fewer bodyparts to focus on each time you visit the gym. Yet because this type of split allows for more sets and higher intensity, it means your muscles will require more rest. Most people who follow an upper/lower split follow a standard Monday (lower-body workout 1), Tuesday (upper-body workout 1), Thursday (lower-body workout 2) and Friday (upper-body workout 2) training schedule as shown. This allows each muscle group two full days of rest between workouts.

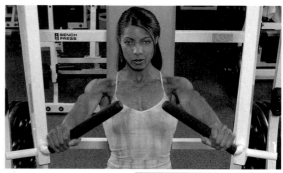

MACHINE CHEST PRESS

MONDAY (LOWER BODY)

BODYPART	EXERCISE	SETS/REPS
Quads/Hams/Glutes	Squat	4/8–10
Quads	Leg Extension	3/12–15
Hamstrings	Lying Leg Curl	3/10–12
Calves	Leg-Press Calf Raise	3/15–20
	Seated Calf Raise	3/20–25
Abs	Hanging Leg Raise	3/10–12
	Crunch	3/15–20

THURSDAY (LOWER BODY)

BODYPART	EXERCISE	SETS/REPS
Quads/Hams/Glutes	Dumbbell Lunge	3/10–12
Hams/Glutes	Romanian Deadlift	3/8–10
Quads	Leg Extension	3/12–15
Calves	Seated Calf Raise	3/15–20
	Standing Calf Raise	3/15–20
Abs	Cable Crunch	3/10–12
	Reverse Crunch	3/15–20

TUESDAY (UPPER BODY)

BODYPART	EXERCISE	SETS/REPS
Chest	Dumbbell Incline Press	3/6–8
	Dumbbell Flye	3/8–10
Back	Lat Pulldown	3/8–10
	Seated Cable Row	3/10–12
Shoulders	Dumbbell Overhead Press	3/8–10
	Lateral Raise	2/12–15
Triceps	Pushdown	2/10–12
	Lying Triceps Extension	2/12–15
Biceps	Barbell Curl	2/10–12
	Preacher Curl	2/12–15

FRIDAY (UPPER BODY)

BODYPART	EXERCISE	SETS/REPS
Back	Barbell Row	3/8–10
	Reverse-Grip Pulldown	3/10–12
Biceps	Dumbbell Incline Curl	2/8–10
	Cable Curl	2/10–12
Chest	Machine Chest Press	3/10–12
	Dumbbell Incline Flye	3/12–15
Shoulders	Upright Row	2/10–12
	Bent-Over Lateral Raise	2/15–20
Triceps	Overhead Triceps Extension	2/8–10
	Kickback	2/10–12

SPLIT NO. 3
Push/Pull/Legs

Three Days Per Week

The push/pull/legs split is based on the concept that the body's muscles are mainly divided into pushing and pulling muscles. Pushing muscles include the chest, shoulders and triceps, which tend to push the weight away from the body such as during the bench press, overhead press and triceps extension. Pulling muscles include the back and biceps, which mainly pull the weight toward the body such as during barbell rows and dumbbell curls. Abs are commonly considered pulling muscles because they pull the torso toward the legs and/or the legs toward the torso.

The problem arises when you consider legs. The squat is a pushing exercise, as is the leg extension, but moves such as leg curls and romanian deadlifts are pulling exercises. But the issue is resolved by giving legs their own training day.

Because the entire body is trained over three separate workouts, many people who follow this split train on Monday, Wednesday and Friday, hitting each muscle group once a week. Yet some do it six days a week to hit each bodypart twice over the seven-day span. We suggest the former to prevent overtraining.

LAT PULLDOWN

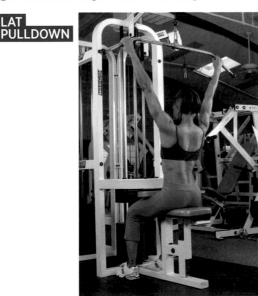

MONDAY (PUSH WORKOUT)

BODYPART	EXERCISE	SETS/REPS
Chest	Bench Press	4/6–8
	Dumbbell Incline Press	4/10–12
	Cable Crossover	4/15–20
Shoulders	Dumbbell Overhead Press	4/8–10
	Lateral Raise	3/12–15
	Reverse Pec-Deck Flye	3/15–20
Triceps	Pushdown	3/10–12
	Lying Triceps Extension	3/12–15
	Overhead Triceps Extension	2/15–20

WEDNESDAY (LEG WORKOUT)

BODYPART	EXERCISE	SETS/REPS
Quads/Hams/Glutes	Dumbbell Lunge	4/6–8
Quads	Leg Press	3/8–10
	Leg Extension	2/12–15
Hams/Glutes	Romanian Deadlift	3/8–10
Hamstrings	Lying Leg Curl	2/10–12
Calves	Standing Calf Raise	3/15–20
	Seated Calf Raise	3/20–25

FRIDAY (PULL WORKOUT)

BODYPART	EXERCISE	SETS/REPS
Back	Dumbbell Row	4/8–10
	Lat Pulldown	4/8–10
	Seated Cable Row	4/10–12
Biceps	Barbell Curl	3/10–12
	Preacher Curl	3/12–15
	Cable Concentration Curl	2/15–20
Abs	Hanging Leg Raise	3/10–12
	Cable Crunch	3/15–20

✳ Bonus Tip
Keep your torso erect at all times — don't lean back excessively — to keep full tension on the upper lats

SPLIT NO. 4

Four-Day

Four Days Per Week

This split simply divides all the major muscle groups of the body into four separate training days. This means you train fewer bodyparts per workout than the three splits we've described, allowing you to increase both the intensity of your workouts, and the number of exercises and sets you perform per muscle group.

Most four-day splits are performed on a Monday, Tuesday, Thursday and Friday schedule, with rest days on Wednesday, Saturday and Sunday. Yet you can train any four days of the week you prefer.

You can divide muscle groups in many ways with a four-day training split, but here we've paired body-parts that perform opposite actions. For example, on Monday you'll train quads, hams, calves and abs; on Tuesday you'll do back and chest; on Thursday you'll work shoulders and abs; and on Friday it's time for biceps and triceps.

The Tuesday and Friday workouts listed here best exemplify the benefits of this training strategy. Pairing chest with back and biceps with triceps allows you to train two muscle groups that don't fatigue each other. Each bodypart performs an opposite motion of its pair, a push vs. a pull.

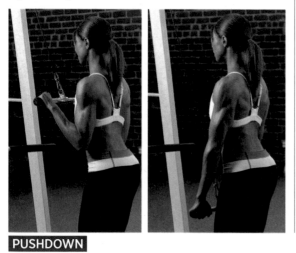

PUSHDOWN

MONDAY (LEGS + ABS)

BODYPART	EXERCISE	SETS/REPS
Quads/Hams/Glutes	Squat	4/8–10
	Step-Up	3/10–15
Quads	Leg Extension	3/12–15
Hamstrings	Lying Leg Curl	3/12–15
Hams/Glutes	Romanian Deadlift	3/12–15
Calves	Standing Calf Raise	4/10–12
	Seated Calf Raise	4/12–15
Abs	Reverse Crunch	3/12–15
	Exercise-Ball Crunch	3/15–20

TUESDAY (BACK + CHEST)

BODYPART	EXERCISE	SETS/REPS
Back	Lat Pulldown	3/8–10
	Barbell Row	3/8–10
	Seated Cable Row	3/10–12
	Straight-Arm Pulldown	3/10–12
Chest	Smith Machine Bench Press	3/8–10
	Dumbbell Incline Press	3/8–10
	Dumbbell Incline Flye	3/10–12
	Pec-Deck or Machine Flye	3/10–12

THURSDAY (SHOULDERS + ABS)

BODYPART	EXERCISE	SETS/REPS
Shoulders	Smith Machine Overhead Press	3/8–10
	Smith Machine Upright Row	3/8–10
	One-Arm Cable Lateral Raise	3/10–12 (each side)
	Bent-Over Lateral Raise	3/10–12
Abs	Decline Crunch	3/12–15
	Oblique Crunch	3/12–15

FRIDAY (BICEPS + TRICEPS)

BODYPART	EXERCISE	SETS/REPS
Biceps	Alternating Dumbbell Curl	3/8–10
	Cable Curl	3/10–12
	EZ-Bar Preacher Curl	3/10–12
Triceps	Smith Machine Close-Grip Bench Press	3/8–10
	Pushdown	3/10–12
	One-Arm Dumbbell Overhead Extension	3/10–12 (each side)

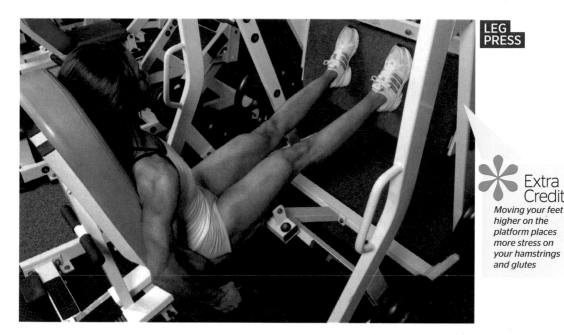

LEG PRESS

✳ Extra Credit
Moving your feet higher on the platform places more stress on your hamstrings and glutes

Splitting the Differences

Follow the program schedule in "Trial Separation" at right, using each training split for three weeks. This will give you just enough time to get a feel for each one and determine how well your body responds, as well as how well it works with your schedule. These are all important considerations. We also give you questions to help you grade the benefits of the various splits.

Regardless of which split you find works best for you, you'll still want to consider swapping it out every once in a while. For example, if you find that the four-day split is your No. 1 choice, use it for a good portion of the year, but every 3–4 months switch to a different training split for at least a month or two.

Trial Separation

This 12-week program lets you put each split through a trial run. Use the workouts listed in the article.

WEEKS	TRAINING SPLIT
1–3	Whole-Body
4–6	Upper/Lower-Body
7–9	Push/Pull/Legs
10–12	Four-Day

Grading the Splits: At the end of 12 weeks, consider the following points.

1) Which split allowed you to train with more intensity and/or provided the best overall results? If you have a well-balanced physique without any weak areas, this is probably the optimal split for you.

2) Which allowed you to train lagging bodyparts the hardest and/or helped bring up lagging areas? If you have a weak bodypart or two that you're trying to raise to the level of the rest of your muscle groups, this split is likely your best option.

3) Which allowed you the best recovery between workouts? If you tend to be sore for days after training and recover slowly, this is the split you should favor.

4) Which was most convenient? If you have a tight schedule and tend to miss workouts because of it, this will probably be the best split for you.

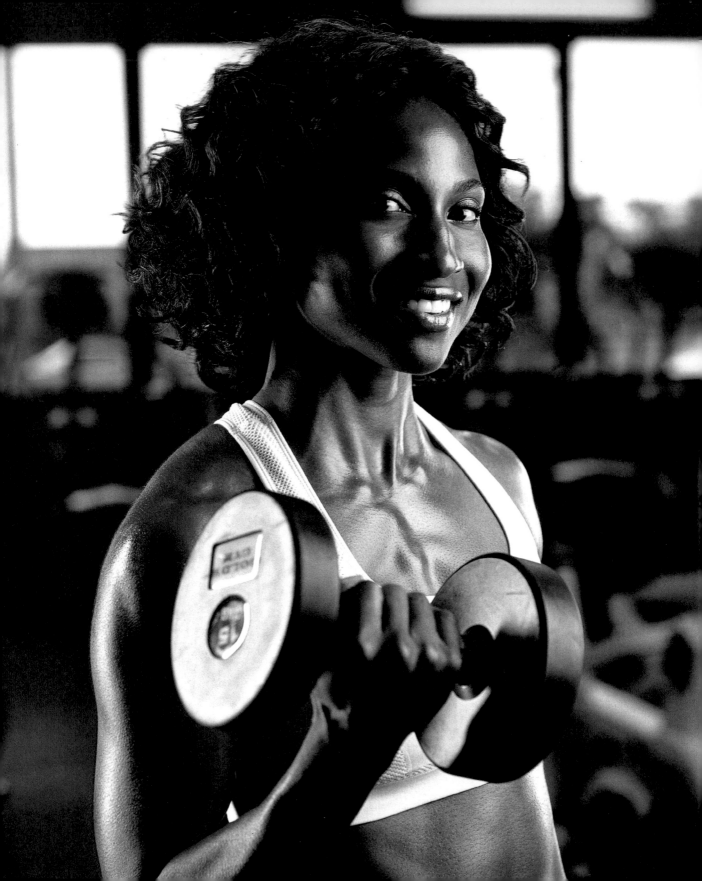

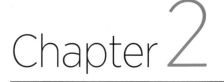

Chapter 2

Fiber *Focus*

Use this six-week program to train all your muscle fibers and achieve the body you desire

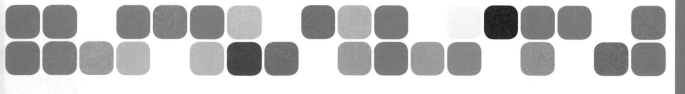

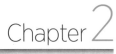
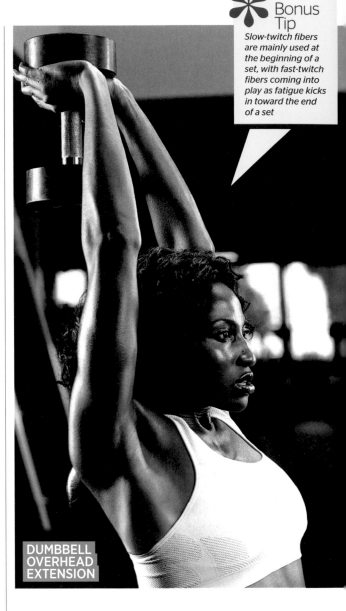

Bonus Tip

Slow-twitch fibers are mainly used at the beginning of a set, with fast-twitch fibers coming into play as fatigue kicks in toward the end of a set

DUMBBELL OVERHEAD EXTENSION

If you were to peel back your skin and look at your muscles, you'd see they appear pretty homogenous. But if you more closely examined what made up this powerful tissue, you'd find it's composed of two types of fibers. Fast-twitch fibers, which help give your muscles shape and size, produce a lot of force and contract quickly, hence their name. They rely on glucose, creatine phosphate and stored adenosine triphosphate (ATP) — your cells' main energy source — to generate explosive high-intensity, short-endurance (anaerobic) activity. They also fatigue easily.

Slow-twitch fibers, on the other hand, help with low force production, contract rather slowly and use fat as their primary source of energy. As such, they generate low-intensity, high-endurance (aerobic) activity. They neither fatigue easily nor grow easily.

Most of us have a 50:50 ratio of fast- to slow-twitch muscle fibers. Some people have a higher percentage of slow-twitch fibers in certain muscles (such as the abs and the soleus, a deep calf muscle), helping them to excel in endurance-type sports such as marathon running and cycling. Other individuals have a higher percentage of fast-twitch fibers in some muscles, which aids them in certain strength and power sports such as weightlifting and track events up to 400 meters.

Stimulating Fibers

But how do we work these fibers? Just picking up a dumbbell to perform a set of biceps curls immediately begins recruiting slow-twitch fibers. Then, as you begin to fatigue during a set, more fast-twitch muscle fibers are recruited. If you take the set to failure or close to it, you'll have successfully trained all the muscle fiber types.

But which kind of muscle fibers should you try to stimulate? Well, using our biceps curl example, there's no way not to train your slow-twitch fibers, so your workout focus really should be on your fast-twitch fibers. That means occasionally using heavy weights, training to failure and/or using fast-rep training methods. So if you typically do 10 reps of biceps curls without breaking a sweat, you need a training paradigm shift. In fact, you should be worried if you don't train with heavy weights from time to time and take your sets to failure — remember, those fast-twitch fibers

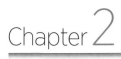

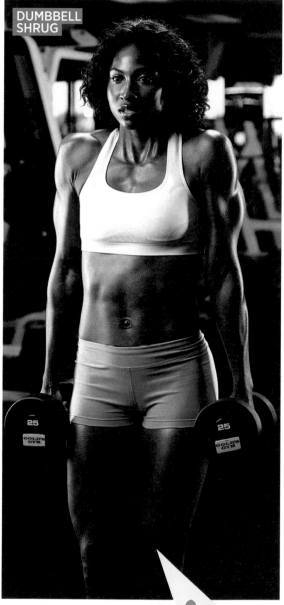

DUMBBELL SHRUG

Week 1

➲ Concentrate on performing 10-rep sets, taking the last set of every exercise to failure.

DAY 1: CHEST + TRICEPS

BODYPART	EXERCISE	SETS	REPS
Chest	Bench Press	3[1]	10
	Dumbbell Incline Press	2	10
	Dumbbell Flye	2	10
Triceps	Pushdown	2[1]	10
	Dumbbell Overhead Extension	2	10
	Dumbbell Kickback	2	10

DAY 2: LEGS + CALVES + ABS

BODYPART	EXERCISE	SETS	REPS
Legs	Squat	3[1]	10
	Leg Press	2	10
	Leg Extension	2	10
	Leg Curl	2	10
	Romanian Deadlift	2[1]	10
Calves	Standing Calf Raise	2	10
	Seated Calf Raise	2	10
Abs	Crunch	2	10
	Reverse Crunch	2	10

DAY 3: REST

DAY 4: SHOULDERS

BODYPART	EXERCISE	SETS	REPS
Shoulders	Barbell Overhead Press	3[1]	10
	Upright Row	2	10
	Dumbbell Lateral Raise	2	10
	Reverse Pec-Deck Flye	2	10

DAY 5: BACK + BICEPS + ABS

BODYPART	EXERCISE	SETS	REPS
Back	Bent-Over Row	3[1]	10
	Lat Pulldown	2	10
	Seated Cable Row	2	10
	Dumbbell Shrug	2	10
Biceps	Barbell Curl	2[1]	10
	Dumbbell Curl	2	10
Abs	Crunch	2	10
	Reverse Crunch	2	10

[1] doesn't include 1–2 warm-up sets of 10–15 reps, not performed to failure

✳ Extra Credit
You'll only develop optimal muscle by using a program that trains both types of muscle fibers

tone and shape your entire body. If you use only light weights and never go heavy or train to failure, then you might never get the physique you want.

For optimal results, you need to work both types of muscle fibers, and our six-week training program can help you do just that. The routines are guaranteed to get you tighter and firmer as well as help you develop more power and strength. Stick with it and you'll be pleased with the changes you see.

The Program

In this program you'll alternate training intensity: Some weeks you'll train with heavier weight, taking your last set of each exercise to muscle failure. Other weeks you'll train with very light weight and fast reps, keeping sets to around five reps each. This will ensure that you're fully working both types of muscle fibers. We've kept the exercises the same each week so you'll become familiar with the routine, allowing you to concentrate fully on each particular rep range. On your heavy-weight weeks, make sure you lift heavy enough to fail at or near the designated rep range. If, for instance, the set calls for 10 reps, don't use a weight with which you could complete, say, 15–20 reps. Using the appropriate resistance is the only way you'll hit those fast-twitch fibers that help you shape a better physique.

Bonus Tip

Take the test on page 20 to find out your own distribution of fast- and slow-twitch muscle fibers

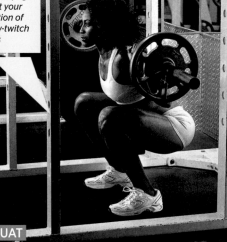

SQUAT

Week 2

↪ Concentrate on explosive reps — less than one second up and less than one second down, five reps per set. Use a weight with which you could complete about 15–20 reps, but stop at five. Exceptions are calves and abs, which tend to have more slow-twitch fibers and don't require explosive training.

DAY 1: CHEST + TRICEPS

BODYPART	EXERCISE	SETS	REPS
Chest	Bench Press	3[1]	5
	Dumbbell Incline Press	2	5
	Dumbbell Flye	2	5
Triceps	Pushdown	2[1]	5
	Dumbbell Overhead Extension	2	5
	Dumbbell Kickback	2	5

DAY 2: LEGS + CALVES + ABS

BODYPART	EXERCISE	SETS	REPS
Legs	Squat	3[1]	5
	Leg Press	2	5
	Leg Extension	2	5
	Leg Curl	2	5
	Romanian Deadlift	2[1]	5
Calves	Seated Calf Raise	3	10
	Standing Calf Raise	3	10
Abs	Crunch	3	10
	Reverse Crunch	3	10

DAY 3: REST

DAY 4: SHOULDERS

BODYPART	EXERCISE	SETS	REPS
Shoulders	Barbell Overhead Press	3[1]	5
	Upright Row	2	5
	Dumbbell Lateral Raise	2	5
	Reverse Pec-Deck Flye	2	5

DAY 5: BACK + BICEPS + ABS

BODYPART	EXERCISE	SETS	REPS
Back	Bent-Over Row	3[1]	5
	Lat Pulldown	2	5
	Seated Cable Row	2	5
	Dumbbell Shrug	2	5
Biceps	Barbell Curl	2[1]	5
	Dumbbell Curl	2	5
Abs	Crunch	3	10
	Reverse Crunch	3	10

[1] doesn't include 1–2 warm-up sets of 10–15 reps, not performed to failure

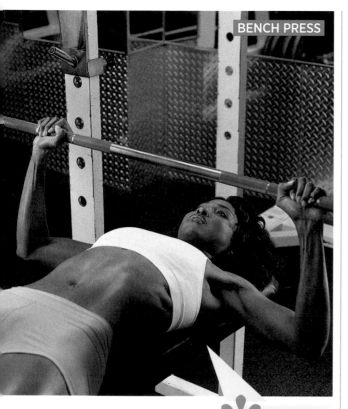

BENCH PRESS

Weeks 3+5

➔ Emphasis on fast-twitch fibers. Concentrate on lifting heavy loads for 10-rep sets, taking the last set of every exercise to failure. Remember to choose a weight that has you reaching failure at 10 reps. If you feel as if you can keep lifting after 10, then the weight isn't heavy enough.

DAY 1: CHEST + TRICEPS

BODYPART	EXERCISE	SETS	REPS
Chest	Bench Press	4[1]	10
	Dumbbell Incline Press	3	10
	Dumbbell Flye	3	10
Triceps	Pushdown	3[1]	10
	Dumbbell Overhead Extension	3	10
	Dumbbell Kickback	3	10

DAY 2: LEGS + CALVES + ABS

BODYPART	EXERCISE	SETS	REPS
Legs	Squat	4[1]	10
	Leg Press	3	10
	Leg Extension	3	10
	Leg Curl	3	10
	Romanian Deadlift	3[1]	10
Calves	Seated Calf Raise	3	10
	Standing Calf Raise	3	10
Abs	Crunch	3	10
	Reverse Crunch	3	10

DAY 3: REST

DAY 4: SHOULDERS

BODYPART	EXERCISE	SETS	REPS
Shoulders	Barbell Overhead Press	4[1]	10
	Upright Row	3	10
	Dumbbell Lateral Raise	3	10
	Reverse Pec-Deck Flye	3	10

DAY 5: BACK + BICEPS + ABS

BODYPART	EXERCISE	SETS	REPS
Back	Bent-Over Row	4[1]	10
	Lat Pulldown	3	10
	Seated Cable Row	3	10
	Dumbbell Shrug	3	10
Biceps	Barbell Curl	3[1]	10
	Dumbbell Curl	3	10
Abs	Crunch	3	10
	Reverse Crunch	3	10

[1] doesn't include 1–2 warm-up sets of 10–15 reps, not performed to failure

✳ Extra Credit

To really give your fast-twitch fibers a workout, you must occasionally train heavy and use fast-rep techniques

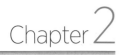
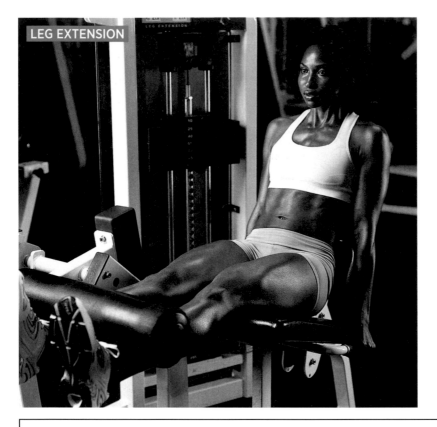

LEG EXTENSION

Fiber Testing

➔ A study from the New York Institute of Technology (Old Westbury) gives us insight into the muscle fibers that make up women's quadriceps. Knowing what type or how much of a certain muscle fiber you have can help give you perspective on your training. To find out where your quads stand on fiber type, you can test them in a similar way.

Step 1) To determine your one-rep max (1RM, the maximum weight you can lift for one and only one rep) on the leg extension, start off by estimating the weight you think you can lift for a single rep only. If you find you can do more than one rep with the weight you selected, rest about three minutes, add 1–2 plates to the weight stack and try again. Do this until you find the weight that allows you to complete one and only one rep.

Step 2) Calculate 70% of your one-rep max. This weight is known as your 70% RM.

Step 3) Do as many reps as you can on the leg extension with your 70% RM.

Step 4) Determine your percentage of fast-twitch fibers:
➔ If you did more than 20 reps, you have less than 50% fast-twitch muscle fibers in your quads. You may excel at running a marathon.
➔ If you did 20 reps, you have about 50% of both fast-twitch and slow-twitch muscle fibers in your quads.
➔ If you did fewer than 20 reps, you have greater than 50% fast-twitch muscle fibers in your quads. You may excel in powerlifting.

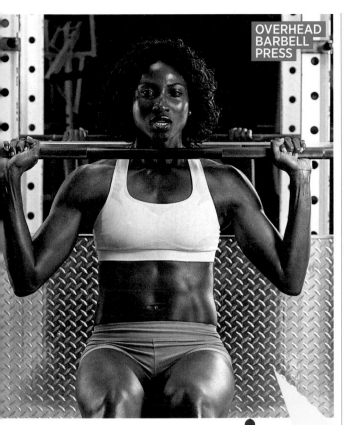

OVERHEAD BARBELL PRESS

Weeks 4+6

➔ Emphasis on slow-twitch fibers. Concentrate on explosive, fast reps. Perform five reps per set at the same speed you used in Week 2. Use a weight with which you can complete about 15–20 reps, but stop at five. Exceptions are calves and abs, which tend to have more slow-twitch fibers and don't require explosive training.

DAY 1: CHEST + TRICEPS

BODYPART	EXERCISE	SETS	REPS
Chest	Bench Press	4[1]	5
	Dumbbell Incline Press	3	5
	Dumbbell Flye	3	5
Triceps	Pushdown	3	5
	Dumbbell Overhead Extension	3	5
	Dumbbell Kickback	3	5

DAY 2: LEGS + CALVES + ABS

BODYPART	EXERCISE	SETS	REPS
Legs	Squat	4[1]	5
	Leg Press	3	5
	Leg Extension	3	5
	Leg Curl	3	5
	Romanian Deadlift	3[1]	5
Calves	Seated Calf Raise	4	10
	Standing Calf Raise	4	10
Abs	Crunch	4	10
	Reverse Crunch	4	10

DAY 3: REST

DAY 4: SHOULDERS

BODYPART	EXERCISE	SETS	REPS
Shoulders	Barbell Overhead Press	4[1]	5
	Upright Row	3	5
	Dumbbell Lateral Raise	3	5
	Reverse Pec-Deck Flye	3	5

DAY 5: BACK + BICEPS + ABS

BODYPART	EXERCISE	SETS	REPS
Back	Bent-Over Row	4[1]	5
	Lat Pulldown	3	5
	Seated Cable Row	3	5
	Dumbbell Shrug	3	5
Biceps	Barbell Curl	3[1]	5
	Dumbbell Curl	3	5
Abs	Crunch	4	10
	Reverse Crunch	4	10

[1] doesn't include 1–2 warm-up sets of 10–15 reps, not performed to failure

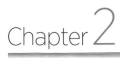

Bonus Tip

The program outlined here will make you tighter and firmer while increasing strength and power

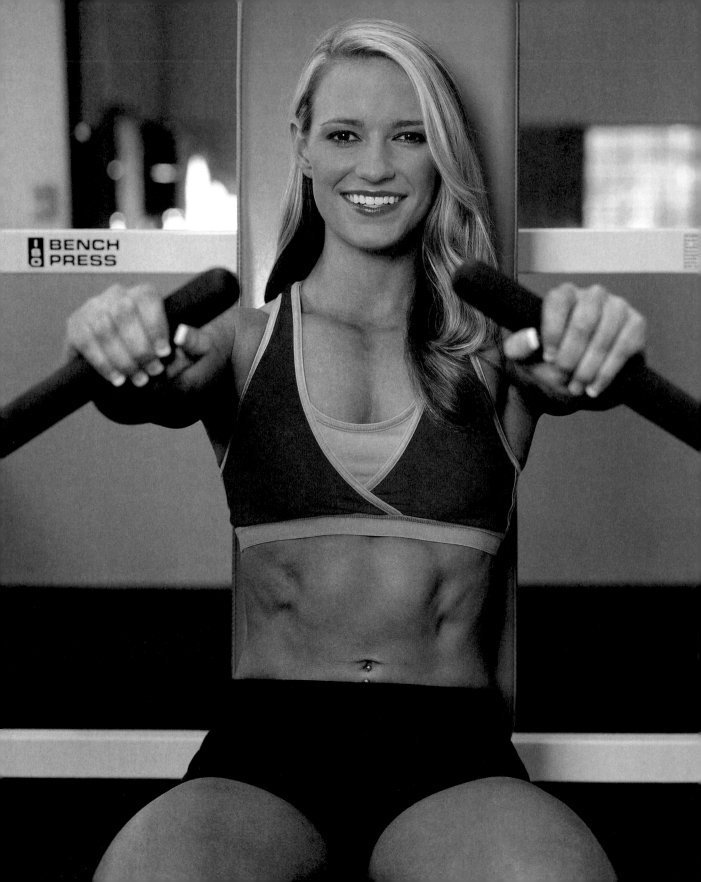

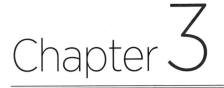

Three Peak

Organize your workouts for optimal muscle-sculpting results with this three-step training plan

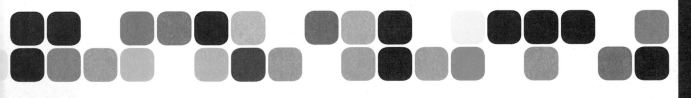

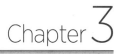 **Walk into any gym and** you'll find a multitude of equipment, from dumbbells and barbells to cable stations and weight machines. Regular M&F HERS readers know the difference between them and how to get a good workout using each. But do you know how to organize your training to maximize the benefits each of these tools offer? You've probably never given it much thought, but there's an order in which you can use each type of equipment to improve your results. We call it "Three-Step Training," and it can help you gain more strength and develop a better physique in three simple steps.

Steady as She Goes

The whole idea behind Three-Step Training centers on the stabilizer muscles. Rather than specifically training the stabilizers, however, this system minimizes stabilizer fatigue so you can maximize the strength and development of your larger bodyparts.

In general, stabilizer muscles (such as the rotator cuffs) lie deep under your major muscle groups (in this case, the delts); the former are typically smaller and weaker than the latter. Yet stabilizer muscles play a critical role in securing the joints during various exercises that larger bodyparts perform. When you reach failure on an exercise, it's often due to stabilizer fatigue and not true fatigue of the major muscle group. When stabilizers are tired, the brain limits nervous system input to the larger muscles to prevent an injury from occurring.

Free-weight and cable exercises require more stabilizer muscle involvement than machine moves. And within the realm of free weights, dumbbell exercises require more stabilizer help than barbell moves. That's because with dumbbells, each arm is allowed to move in all directions at the shoulder joint, whereas with barbell exercises the arms can move in fewer directions because both hands are fixed on the bar. Among cable exercises, one-arm moves (such as the one-arm seated row for back) call on more stabilizers than two-arm cable exercises (such as the wide-grip seated row). Finally, machines (which include the Smith machine and selectorized weight machines) require very little stabilizer involvement since they follow a predetermined path that doesn't permit deviation.

Thus, the order of involvement of the stabilizer

Stepping Stones

↪ Try these sample three-step workouts for each major muscle group. Work them into your usual training split, or try our recommended split of chest and shoulders on Mondays, back and abs on Tuesdays, thighs and calves on Thursdays, and arms and abs on Fridays. (For abs and calves, use a standard program; the three steps aren't overly beneficial to these two bodyparts.)

EXERCISE	SETS	REPS
CHEST		
Dumbbell Bench Press	3	8–10
Barbell Incline Press	3	8–10
Pec-Deck Flye	3	12–15
SHOULDERS		
Seated Dumbbell Overhead Press	3	8–10
Barbell Upright Row	3	8–10
Machine Lateral Raise	3	12–15
BACK		
One-Arm Dumbbell Row	3	8–10 (each side)
Wide-Grip Pulldown	3	8–10
Machine Seated Row	3	12–15
LEGS		
Dumbbell Step-Up	3	8–10
Barbell Squat	3	8–10
Leg Press	3	8–10
Leg Extension	3	12–15
Lying Leg Curl	3	12–15
TRICEPS		
One-Arm Reverse-Grip Pushdown	2	8–10 (each side)
Lying Triceps Extension	2	8–10
Machine Triceps Extension	2	12–15
BICEPS		
Dumbbell Incline Curl	2	8–10
Cable Curl	2	8–10
Machine Preacher Curl	2	12–15

CONCENTRATION CURL

TARGET: *Biceps*

GET READY: *Sit at the end of a bench, lean forward at the hips and support yourself with one hand on the same-side knee. Grasp a dumbbell and brace your working elbow against the same-side inner thigh.*

GO: *Curl the weight toward your upper chest. Pause a few inches away, then lower the dumbbell along the same arc back to the start. Repeat for reps, then switch sides.*

✻ Bonus Tip

Keep your elbow pressed against your inner thigh throughout the movement and avoid rounding your back

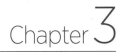

BENCH PRESS

TARGET: *Chest*
GET READY: *Lie faceup on a bench, feet flat on the floor. Grasp the bar with your hands slightly wider than shoulder-width apart.*
GO: *Lift the bar off the rack, then bend your elbows to bring it to your lower chest. Forcefully push the bar back up to the start, stopping just short of elbow lockout.*

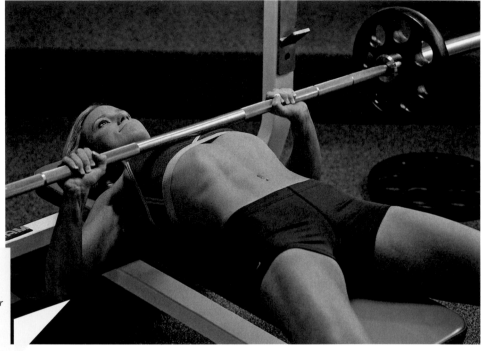

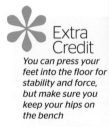
Extra Credit
You can press your feet into the floor for stability and force, but make sure you keep your hips on the bench

muscles from most to least goes 1) dumbbells and one-arm cable exercises, 2) barbells and two-arm cable moves, and 3) machines. By performing exercises that require more stabilizer involvement earlier in your workout and moves that require less stabilizer involvement later, you can more effectively train your major muscle groups. This leads to superior gains in strength and development in a shorter period.

Step Into It

With the Three-Step Training program, each step of your workout progresses to a different type of training, each of which incurs less impact on the stabilizers. This allows you to optimally train the larger muscle groups without the stabilizers limiting your intensity later in the session.

➔ **Step 1** is a dumbbell or one-arm cable exercise; because these moves require more stabilizer help, do them when your stabilizers are strongest.

➔ **Step 2** is a barbell or two-arm cable exercise, which require less stabilizer involvement than the Step 1 movement.

MACHINE SEATED ROW

TARGET: *Back*
GET READY: *Place your feet on the footrests and your chest flush against the pad, arching your back slightly. Grasp the handles using a close, neutral grip; this keeps your elbows near your sides, which places more stress on your lower lats.*
GO: *Pull the handles toward you and squeeze your back muscles. Pause, then slowly return to the start.*

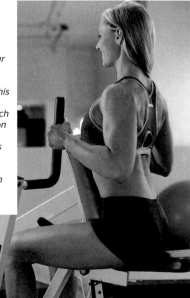

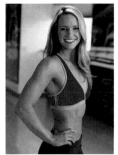

Step Substitutes

Try swapping these exercises into your Three-Step Training program:

BODYPART	STEP 1 EXERCISES	STEP 2 EXERCISES	STEP 3 EXERCISES

CHEST	Dumbbell Press (flat, incline or decline)
	Dumbbell Flye (flat, incline or decline)
	Cable Flye (flat, incline or decline)
		Bench Press
		  (flat, incline or decline)
		Dip
		Push-Up
			Machine Chest Press
			Machine Flye
			Pec-Deck Flye
			Smith Machine Bench Press
			  (flat, incline or decline)

SHOULDERS	Dumbbell Overhead Press Dumbbell Lateral Raise Dumbbell Front Raise Dumbbell Bent-Over Lateral Raise Dumbbell Upright Row Cable Lateral Raise One-Arm Cable Front Raise One-Arm Cable Overhead Press	Barbell Overhead Press Barbell Front Raise Barbell Upright Row	Machine Overhead Press Smith Machine Overhead Press Machine Lateral Raise Smith Machine Upright Row Reverse Pec-Deck Flye
BACK	One-Arm Dumbbell Row One-Arm Cable Row One-Arm Lat Pulldown	Barbell Row Lat Pulldown Pull-Up Seated Cable Row Decline Pullover	Machine Seated Row Smith Machine Row Machine Lat Pulldown Machine Pullover
LEGS	Barbell or Dumbbell Lunge One-Leg Squat Barbell or Dumbbell Step-Up One-Leg Romanian Deadlift	Squat Dumbbell Squat Romanian Deadlift	Leg Press Smith Machine Squat Smith Machine Front Squat Hack Squat Leg Extension Leg Curl (lying, seated or standing)

TRICEPS	One-Arm Dumbbell Overhead Extension
	One-Arm Pushdown
	  (overhand or underhand grip)
	Kickback (dumbbell or cable)
	Dumbbell Lying Triceps Extension
	Dumbbell Close-Grip Bench Press
		Close-Grip Bench Press
		Pushdown
		Lying Triceps Extension
		  (barbell, EZ-bar or cable)
		Overhead Triceps
		  Extension
		Bench Dip
			Triceps Extension Machine
			Dip Machine
			Smith Machine Close-Grip
			  Bench Press
			Machine Chest Press
			  (with close/neutral grip)

BICEPS	Dumbbell Curl (standing or seated) Incline Curl (dumbbell or cable) Concentration Curl (dumbbell or cable) One-Arm Cable Curl Dumbbell Preacher Curl	Barbell Curl EZ-Bar Curl Cable Curl Cable Preacher Curl	Machine Curl Machine Preacher Curl Smith Machine Drag Curl

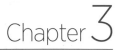
SEATED CABLE ROW

TARGET: *Back*
GET READY: *Sit at a cable-row station with your back straight and your knees slightly bent. Grasp the handles using a neutral grip.*
GO: *Squeeze your shoulder blades together, then bend your elbows and pull with your middle-back muscles to bring the handle to your midsection. Keep your back tight and erect, and your arms close to your sides throughout the move.*

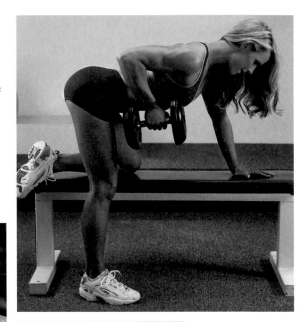

ONE-ARM DUMBBELL ROW

TARGET: *Back*
GET READY: *Place one knee and the same-side hand on a bench so your torso is roughly parallel to the floor. Grasp a dumbbell in your free hand using a neutral grip, arm extended toward the floor. Keep your back tight and arched throughout the movement.*
GO: *Bend your elbow to pull the weight up and slightly toward your hip. Squeeze your lat, then slowly return to the start. Repeat for reps, then switch sides.*

➲ **Step 3** is a machine exercise, which targets the major muscle and involves hardly any stabilizers.

As an example of a three-step workout for shoulders, you could do three sets of seated dumbbell overhead presses followed by three sets of barbell upright rows and three sets of machine lateral raises. (For more sample workouts, see "Stepping Stones" on page 24; for a list of alternate exercises, see "Step Substitutes" on page 27.)

Getting a Leg Up

Before you head to the gym, let's clear up the issue of leg training as it relates to the Three-Step philosophy. Starting with dumbbell or unilateral cable exercises for legs just doesn't apply. The key to Step 1 is allowing each limb to work independently. For legs, simply

choose a one-leg exercise for Step 1. This has the same effect as using dumbbells for upper-body muscle groups: involvement of more stabilizer muscles.

In Step 2 for legs, choose a two-leg free-weight exercise. This has the same effect as barbell or two-arm cable moves for upper body: It involves less stabilizer use than Step 1 moves but more than those of Step 3.

Finally, for Step 3 choose a machine squatting type of exercise (such as a leg press or hack squat), as well as leg-extension and leg-curl machines. Yes, legs require more exercises because you're training two muscle groups — quads and hamstrings.

Now, if you're ready for a novel challenge in the gym, formulate your plan of attack, either using our sample routines or creating one of your own. It could prove to be just the three steps you need to drastically improve your body.

MACHINE PREACHER CURL

TARGET: *Biceps*
GET READY: *Adjust the seat so your armpits are flush with the top of the pad. Use an underhand, shoulder-width grip and bend your elbows slightly.*
GO: *Curl the handles until your forearms are about perpendicular to the floor. Pause, then return to the start. Don't allow your elbows to flare out as you perform the movement.*

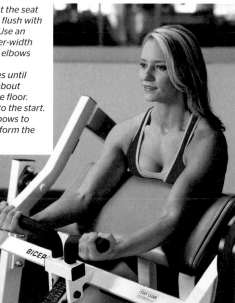

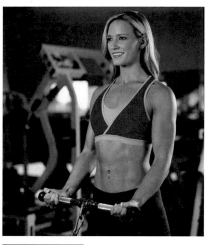

CABLE CURL

TARGET: *Biceps*
GET READY: *Attach a straight bar to a low-pulley cable and use a shoulder-width, underhand grip. Take a step back from the weight stack.*
GO: *Keeping your shoulders down and back, slowly curl the bar toward your shoulders. Pause, then reverse the motion, stopping just short of full-arm extension at the bottom.*

DUMBBELL BENCH PRESS

TARGET: *Chest*
GET READY: *Lie faceup on a flat bench with your feet on the floor. Grasp a pair of dumbbells and hold them outside your shoulders, elbows bent about 90 degrees.*
GO: *Press the weights over your chest so they almost touch without locking out your elbows. Squeeze your chest hard; don't relax in the top position.*

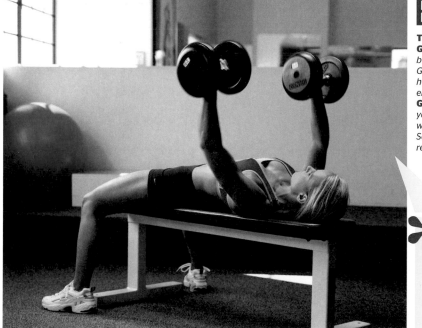

Bonus Tip

Dumbbells require more balance to control than a barbell, so consider using lighter weights at first

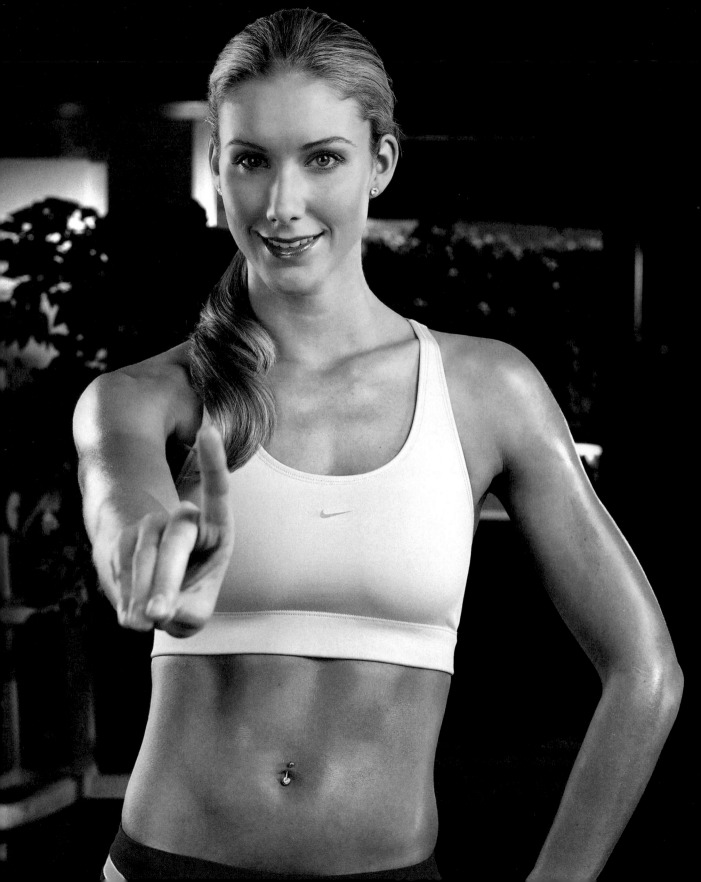

Single Minded

Unilateral training can help you become stronger and more defined, one limb at a time

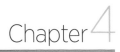

Atop the long list of often-used but little-understood exercise variables stands unilateral training, wherein you work just one muscle or limb independently of the opposite side. Maybe you find yourself diligently grinding out rep after rep of a single-leg press or a one-arm dumbbell curl without giving much thought as to why. But unilateral training is far more than a thoughtless trend or fashionable gym pastime. It's one of the most effective ways to elicit change from stubborn or lagging muscle groups and can add productive variety to your stale routine. So get ready to find out why you should put your best foot (or other limb of choice) forward in the gym — this time, with purpose.

One-Sided Argument

Bilateral training, in which you train both sides of a bodypart (such as arms, chest, delts, quads, calves, etc.) simultaneously, is the more traditional approach to exercise selection. Unilateral training, however, offers a number of advantages over its bilateral counterpart, including snuffing out strength and physique imbalances, as well as increasing core engagement.

Most of us are stronger on one side than the other; for example, the right arm and leg are usually stronger on a right-handed person. Thus, training one side or limb at a time encourages more balance between your right and left sides, both in terms of power and muscular development. A person who curls a 40-pound barbell for 10 reps, for instance, may find that one arm can curl 25 pounds comfortably while the other can handle only 15 or 20 pounds on its own. Unilateral training allows you to take the dominant side out of the equation, isolating the weaker side and thus forcing it to become stronger and/or more developed.

"Training this way also results in greater joint and core stabilization," says Johanna Spates, a certified personal trainer and performance enhancement specialist (PES) at 360 Sports Performance in Reseda, California. "You cannot negate unilateral training's impact on the core because several muscles are activated in a stabilizing role."

She also points out that many day-to-day movements — from opening a door to grabbing a gallon of milk out of the refrigerator — are done unilaterally with a favored arm, making it stronger. Therefore,

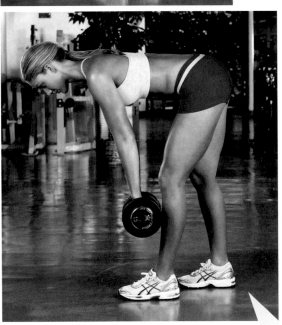

Bonus Tip
By staggering your feet, this move directs the tension to the glute and hamstring of your forward leg

ONE-LEG ROMANIAN DEADLIFT

TARGETS: *Glutes, hamstrings*
GET READY: *Stand holding dumbbells alongside your thighs, back slightly arched. Stagger your feet just inside shoulder width and bend your knees slightly.*
GO: *Maintaining the slight arch in your back, push your glutes back and lean forward at the hips until you feel a stretch in your hamstrings. Pause, then squeeze your glutes and hams to return to the start. Make sure both weights stay close to your front leg throughout the move. Repeat for reps, then switch sides.*

Extra Credit
Raise your back leg straight behind you while squeezing your glutes

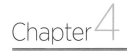

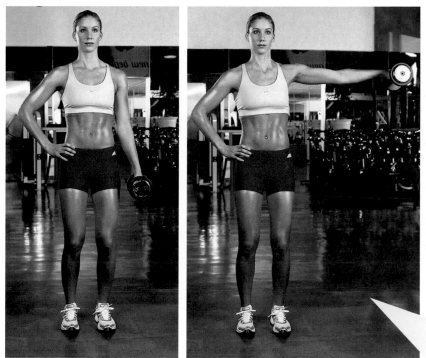

STANDING ONE-ARM LATERAL RAISE

TARGET: *Shoulders*
GET READY: *Stand holding a dumbbell at your side with a slight bend in your elbow. Place your nonworking hand on your hip.*
GO: *With your back straight and your knees slightly bent, raise the weight out to your side in a wide arc to shoulder level. Squeeze your delt hard and return to the start. Repeat for reps, then switch sides.*

 Bonus Tip

For added intensity, stop the dumbbell about 6 inches from your hip on the return. You can also use a D-handle attached to a low-pulley cable, grasping the handle in your outside hand

unilateral training — in which you submit your inherently weaker side to the same workload as the stronger side — is all the more relevant.

Research shows that unilateral training also helps you work more total muscle fibers than you would with traditional, two-sided exercises. A 2003 study from *The Journals of Gerontology Series A: Biological Sciences & Medical Sciences* reported that the force generated on a two-arm barbell curl was up to 20% less than the sum of the force produced from the left- and right-arm unilateral dumbbell curls. "In a unilateral exercise, muscles will recruit more force-producing, fast-twitch fibers to offset the fact that fewer overall fibers contribute to the movement," says Michele Olson, PhD, FACSM, CSCS, professor of exercise science at Auburn University at Montgomery (Alabama). For instance, when curling with your right arm, that biceps must recruit more of its own fast-twitch fibers than it would for a two-handed curl since it receives no help from the left biceps.

In addition, Rodney Corn, MA, PES, CSCS, director of education at the National Academy of Sports Medicine (NASM), points out: "Physiologically, [uni-lateral training] can require higher levels of core activation to maintain balance while working one side and not the other." That equates to more work for your abs and lower back without yet another day of crunches and Russian twists. And its superior core activation means unilateral training is a welcome change of pace for those who typically don't lift this way.

Know Thyself

Clearly, unilateral training has a number of advantages that might warrant using it more often, but — you knew there was a "but" coming, right? — consider these factors before diving into a unilateral program:

➔ **It can be too advanced for beginners.** "People may try to get too fancy with the exercises or go too heavy and lose the benefits because they must compensate by cheating or bouncing," Corn says. Unseasoned lifters should experiment with lighter loads to master unilateral moves and progress injury-free.

➔ **It can be time-intensive.** Doing three sets of one-arm triceps pushdowns will take twice as long (six sets total) as its two-arm counterpart. So those wanting to

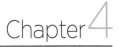

Bonus Tip

Avoid using momentum. Use a slow, controlled pace to maximize intensity and avoid injury

train this way must be able to see the payoff ahead and be willing to sacrifice the time it takes to get there.

➔ **It's not for those whose attention wanders.** Unilateral trainees must also be keenly observant of their own weaknesses to determine proper loads and lifting volume. Training your weaker side with too little weight or volume can result in a persistent imbalance, so constantly challenge yourself to bring up any that you notice. On the other hand, training with too much weight or volume on one side can result in overtraining of the muscle, regardless of your strength.

➔ **If you want to gain strength,** train unilaterally early in your workout. Since these moves often require more stability, it's best to do them when you're fresh and can exert the most force, which is key to handling greater loads and getting stronger. If you want to dial in muscle definition, train unilaterally late or last in your workout. High-rep, one-sided moves can provide an excellent pump at the end of your session.

"As is the case with any training regimen, unilateral training shouldn't be used solely or without variation to avoid plateaus in progress," Corn says. The smarter approach might be to sprinkle one or two unilateral moves into your current program, switching them up occasionally to prevent your body from getting used to a particular routine.

STANDING ONE-ARM CABLE CROSSOVER

TARGET: *Chest*
GET READY: *Grasp a D-handle attached to a high-pulley cable in one hand and step away from the stack so your arm extends out to your side at shoulder level. Place your nonworking hand on your hip.*
GO: *Keeping your knees and working arm slightly bent and your back straight, pull the handle across your body toward your opposite hip in a wide arc. Hold the peak contraction, then slowly return to the start. Repeat for reps, then switch sides.*

Extra Credit

In this one-arm version, don't stagger your stance; keep your feet square and a bit wider apart than normal to aid your balance

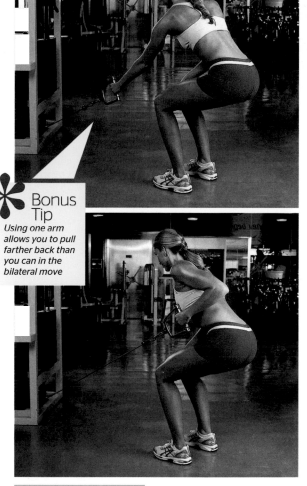

Bonus Tip

Using one arm allows you to pull farther back than you can in the bilateral move

STANDING ONE-ARM CABLE ROW

TARGET: *Back*
GET READY: *Grasp a D-handle attached to a low-pulley cable using a neutral grip. Step back, then bend your knees and lean forward at the hips. Fully extend your working arm.*
GO: *Keeping your head neutral and back slightly arched, bring the handle to your side by pulling your elbow back as far as possible without twisting your torso. Squeeze your back before resisting the weight's return to the start. Repeat for reps, then switch sides.*

One-Sided Training Guide

➔ This approach will have you training unilaterally throughout each session, adding serious variety to your workouts. Try these bodypart routines for four weeks each, or use them occasionally to change up your current program. Alternate which side you begin unilateral exercises with from workout to workout, which leads to greater balance. Select weights that allow you to fail at the designated rep range.

TARGET: LEGS

EXERCISE	SETS/REPS
Leg Press	3/10
One-Leg Romanian Deadlift	2/12 (each side)
Romanian Deadlift	2/10
Leg Curl	3/12
Leg Extension	3/12
One-Leg Extension	2/10 (each side)

TARGET: CHEST

EXERCISE	SETS/REPS
Bench Press	3/12
Standing One-Arm Cable Crossover	3/12 (each side)
Cable Crossover	2/10
Dumbbell Bench Press	3/12
One-Arm Dumbbell Bench Press	2/10 (each side)
Push-Up	3/failure[1]

[1] Perform as many reps as you can, resting no more than 90 seconds between sets.

TARGET: BACK

EXERCISE	SETS/REPS
Barbell Row	3/12
One-Arm Dumbbell Row	2/10 (each side)
Standing Cable Row	3/12
Standing One-Arm Cable Row	2/10 (each side)
One-Arm Lat Pulldown	2/10 (each side)
Front Pulldown	3/12

TARGET: SHOULDERS

EXERCISE	SETS/REPS
Dumbbell Overhead Press	3/12
One-Arm Dumbbell Overhead Press	2/10 (each side)
Standing Lateral Raise	3/12
Standing One-Arm Lateral Raise	2/10 (each side)
Bent-Over Lateral Raise	3/12

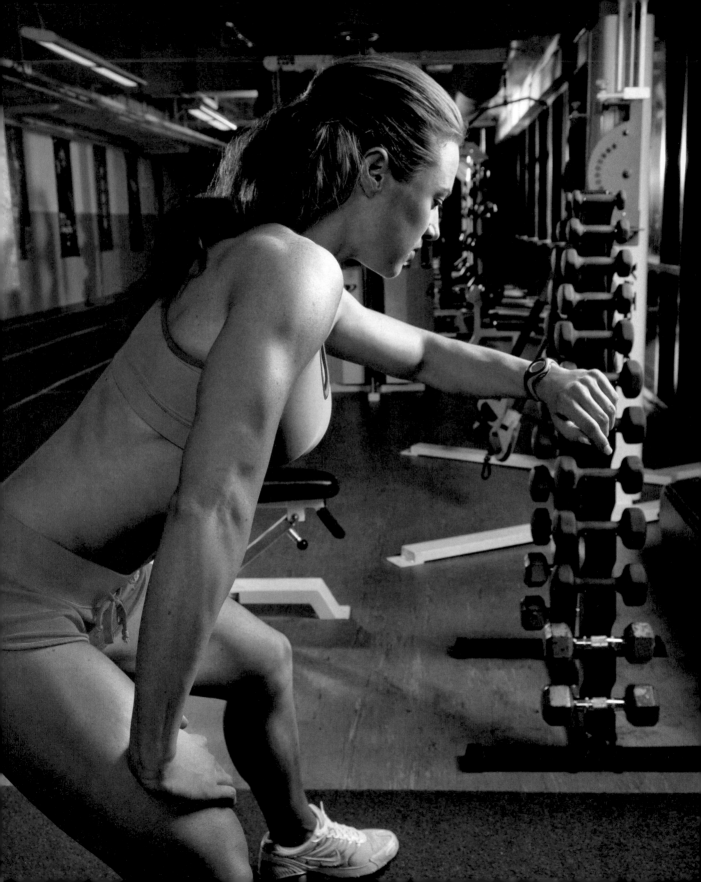

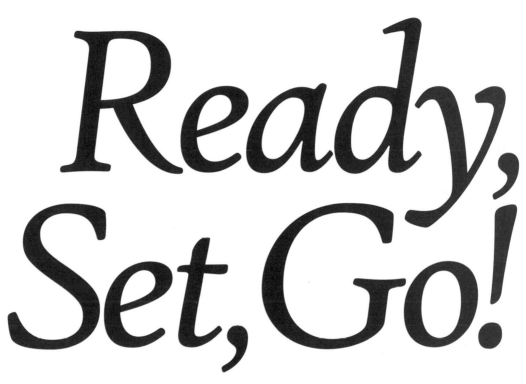

Chapter 5

Ready, Set, Go!

*Crunched for time? No worries.
These five 30-minute routines are
short on time but long on results*

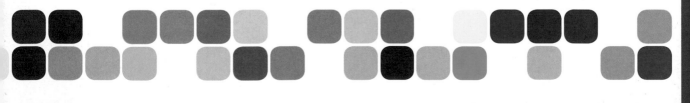

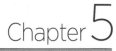
Sure, it would be great if everyone had an hour or two every day to commit to fitness. Heck, finding that time could be downright easy if you didn't have to go to work, take care of family obligations, run errands and sleep. You may feel as if your quest for a fitter body might get squeezed out of your schedule altogether.

Good news: It doesn't have to be. Don't have 60–90 minutes to spend at the gym? No problem, because we've crammed everything you need into a selection of five potent 30-minute workouts. These ultra-efficient sessions are high on intensity, low on rest, and packed with proven exercises and welcome variety, making them fun and effective.

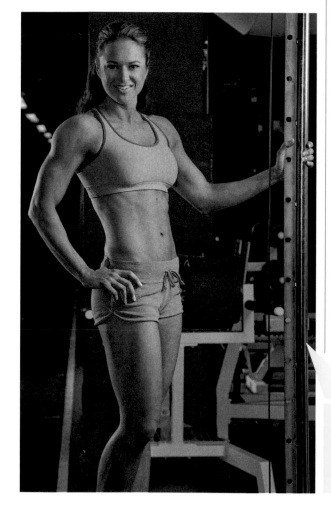

● Even if you have only 30 minutes a day to train, you can still achieve your goals in the gym with the right training program

Workout No. 1
Legs & Shoulders

➲ A goal of this workout is to enhance the illusion of a smaller waist by adding some curves to your shoulders. Why are legs in the mix? For one, they work independently of the delts, so you don't have to worry about overfatiguing one bodypart as the workout progresses. Second, shoulders are a relatively small muscle group, so incorporating legs into the routine greatly increases the amount of calories you can burn.

30-MINUTE METHODS: SUPERSETS, HIGH REPS, VARIETY

EXERCISE	SETS	REPS
Dumbbell Squat	2	20
— superset with —		
Dumbbell Overhead Press	2	20
Leg Extension	2	20
— superset with —		
Cable Front Raise	2	20
Leg Curl	2	20
— superset with —		
Lateral Raise	2	20
Cable Lunge	2	20
— superset with —		
Reverse Pec-Deck Flye	2	20
Wall Squat With Static Lateral Raise	4	to failure

NOTE: During all supersets, rest only as long as it takes to set up for the next exercise. Rest as little as possible — no longer than 45 seconds — between all working sets.

CABLE FRONT RAISE

TARGET: *Shoulders*
GET READY: *Stand erect facing away from a low-pulley cable station with dual pulleys, grasping a D-handle in each hand using an overhand grip. Begin with your arms extended at your sides.*
GO: *Keeping your arms straight, raise the handles in front of you to just above parallel to the floor. Squeeze your shoulders at the top, then slowly return to the start.*

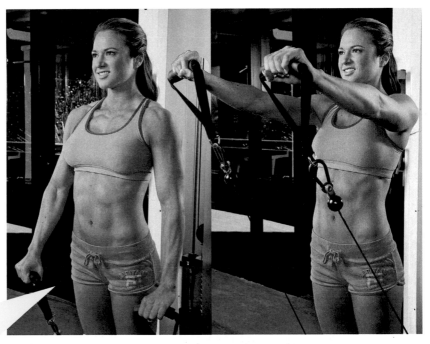

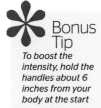

Bonus Tip

To boost the intensity, hold the handles about 6 inches from your body at the start

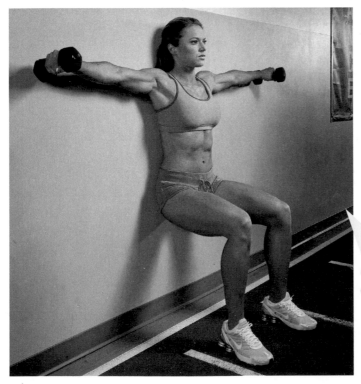

WALL SQUAT WITH STATIC LATERAL RAISE

TARGETS: *Quads, shoulders*
GET READY: *Grasp a pair of light dumbbells and stand with your hips and back flush against a wall, feet shoulder-width apart in front of you.*
GO: *Bend your knees to slide down the wall, descending until your knees form 90-degree angles as you simultaneously raise the weights out to your sides in an arc to shoulder level. Hold both positions as long as possible, then return to the start.*

Extra Credit

If your shoulders fail first, drop the dumbbells and continue squatting

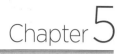
30-Minute Methods

Each of these routines uses several tactics to increase intensity and elicit more benefit in less time. Try them as prescribed and continue experimenting with them in your regular workouts.

➔ **Constant Tension** While using free weights is best for getting stronger and leaner in the gym, they're not without weakness. Some exercises, such as the preacher curl, have "holes" in the movement where it becomes temporarily easier. Cables, however, keep tension on the muscle throughout the move, making them a good choice for quick, effective workouts.

➔ **Compound Movements** These multijoint exercises — such as the bench press, squat and lat pulldown — call on several different muscle groups, meaning you'll break down more muscle fibers than with single-joint moves. Your body's efforts to repair itself burns more calories and you'll come back stronger. Any routine should revolve around these types of exercises.

➔ **High Reps** High-rep sets not only leave your muscles feeling tight but also provide a higher calorie burn during a workout. High-rep (12 or more) sets also build muscular endurance and athletic performance. Keep your rest periods short (30–45 seconds) for an even greater burn.

➔ **Low Reps** Heavier sets (6–8 reps) build strength that's ideal for long-term physique changes and, when paired with shorter rest periods, actually provide a greater increase in your resting metabolic rate for longer after a workout.

➔ **100s** While 100 reps in a set seems unfathomable, this type of training taps into every available muscle fiber in a given set. You'll do them here only for calf raises, but 100s training can be applied to nearly any exercise using a weight that's about 20% of your one-rep max. Aim to complete up to 70 reps nonstop, then rest for as many seconds as the number of reps you have remaining. Repeat this pattern until you reach 100 reps. One set per muscle group is plenty, making it perfect when you need to complete as much work in as short a time as possible.

➔ **Variety of Exercises** Incorporating unfamiliar movements into your routine places a greater demand on your target muscles. By tapping into underused muscle fibers, you enhance your overall muscle quality. Mastering new moves also develops greater mind-muscle coordination.

Workout No. 2
Back, Hamstrings & Glutes

➔ You want to look just as good walking out of a room as you do walking in. That means paying due attention to your back, hamstrings and glutes. Not surprisingly, these are among many people's least favorite bodyparts to train. The lifts require a lot of muscle and demand a great deal of energy. But hey, if you can crank through a killer routine for all these major muscle groups in just 30 minutes, then it becomes a lot more palatable, right?

30-MINUTE METHODS: COMPOUND MOVEMENTS, LOW REPS, HIGH REPS, VARIETY

EXERCISE	SETS	REPS
Assisted Pull-Up	1	20–30¹
Leg Curl	1	20–30¹
Back Extension	1	20–30¹
Romanian Deadlift	3	8–10
Cable Glute-Ham Raise	2	10–12
Cable Straight-Leg Kickback	2	12–15 (each side)
Seated Row	2	15–20
Assisted Pull-Up	1	to failure

¹ warm-up set — do not take to failure

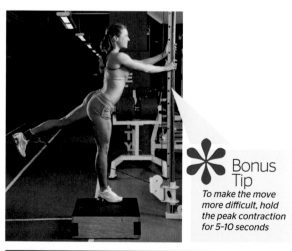

Bonus Tip
To make the move more difficult, hold the peak contraction for 5–10 seconds

CABLE STRAIGHT-LEG KICKBACK

TARGET: *Glutes*
GET READY: *Attach an ankle cuff to a low-pulley cable. Affix the cuff to one ankle and lean slightly forward to grasp the machine for support. If possible, stand on a short box or platform.*
GO: *Keeping your abs tight, bring your working leg as far forward as you can without letting the weight stack touch down. Contract your glutes and hamstrings, and drive through your heel to pull your leg behind you. Repeat for reps, then switch sides.*

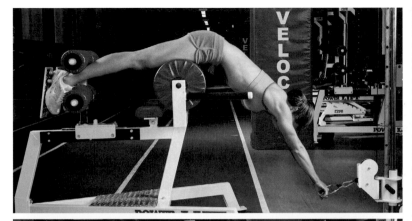

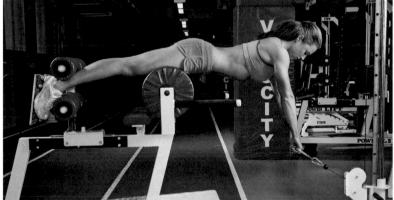

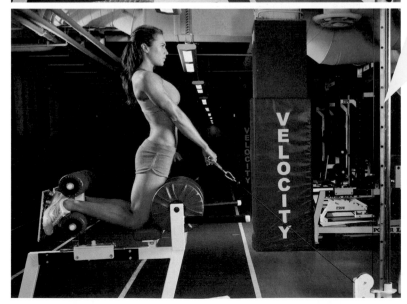

CABLE GLUTE-HAM RAISE

TARGETS: *Back, glutes, hamstrings*

GET READY: *Place a back-extension bench near a low-pulley cable. Position your ankles under the rollers and your thighs against the pad. Grasp the D-handle with both hands and begin with your torso at about a 45-degree angle to the floor.*

GO: *Pull yourself up using your hams and glutes until your body is straight from heels to head. Continue pulling yourself up slowly by bending your knees, raising your torso until it's perpendicular to the floor.*

❋ Extra Credit

A strong glute-ham region provides a powerful training foundation by helping to stabilize your body

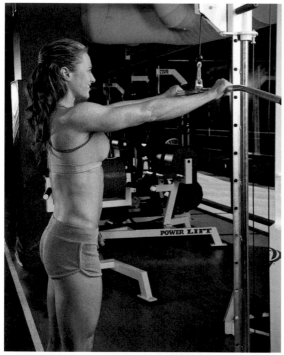

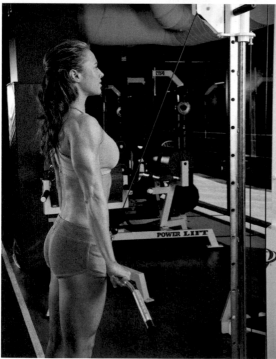

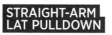

Workout No. 3
Upper Body & Abs

⊃ Although you want a stronger-looking upper body, you just don't have enough time (or days in the week) to devote to chest, back, shoulders, biceps, triceps and abs. Or do you? This routine, which employs similar movement patterns within supersets, puts all of those muscle groups to the test in a very short amount of time. (Note: You could complete this workout in about 15 minutes!) Every superset works through a similar plane in push/pull fashion — for example, a lat pulldown followed by an overhead press. Training opposing muscle groups back to back helps you stay strong throughout the routine, which is why this type of superset is a great idea for the time-crunched masses.

30-MINUTE METHODS: SUPERSETS, COMPOUND MOVEMENTS

EXERCISE	SETS	REPS
Lat Pulldown	2	12
— superset with —		
Overhead Press	2	12
Cable Front Raise	2	12
— superset with —		
Straight-Arm Lat Pulldown	2	12
Wide-Grip Seated Row	2	12
— superset with —		
Machine Chest Press	2	12
Cable Curl	2	12
— superset with —		
Rope Pushdown	2	12
Double Crunch	2	to failure

STRAIGHT-ARM LAT PULLDOWN

TARGET: *Back*
GET READY: *Stand erect facing a weight stack using a shoulder-width stance. Grasp the bar using an overhand grip, hands shoulder-width apart. Begin with the bar at shoulder level, arms extended.*
GO: *Pull the bar toward your thighs in a wide arc, focusing on using just your lats. Squeeze your lats hard, then return to the start in a smooth, controlled motion.*

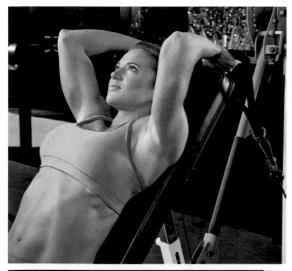

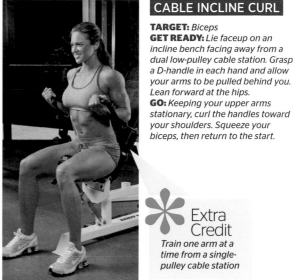

CABLE INCLINE CURL

TARGET: *Biceps*
GET READY: *Lie faceup on an incline bench facing away from a dual low-pulley cable station. Grasp a D-handle in each hand and allow your arms to be pulled behind you. Lean forward at the hips.*
GO: *Keeping your upper arms stationary, curl the handles toward your shoulders. Squeeze your biceps, then return to the start.*

✳ Extra Credit
Train one arm at a time from a single-pulley cable station

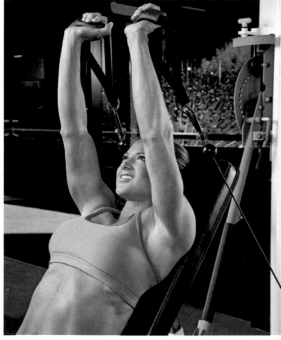

CABLE INCLINE TRICEPS EXTENSION

TARGET: *Triceps*
GET READY: *Lie faceup on an incline bench facing away from a dual low-pulley cable station. Grasp a D-handle in each hand. Keep your feet flat on the floor.*
GO: *With your arms bent and elbows near your head, keep your upper arms stationary as you press the handles toward the ceiling. Squeeze your tri's hard, then slowly return to the start.*

Workout No. 4
Arms, Calves & Abs

➲ Instead of running around the gym looking for the right set of dumbbells or moving from one machine to the next, try staying put for a change. This all-cable workout, which eliminates the need to switch stations, is perfect for hitting your arms, calves and abs. Plus, cables offer constant tension, which heavily taxes your muscles throughout the range of motion. To further exhaust the targeted muscles, extend the last set of each exercise by reducing the weight and continuing to failure. And for your calves, we have something sinister: one set of 100 reps. Yes, it's okay to use just your bodyweight for this monster set.

30-MINUTE METHODS:
LOW REPS, CONSTANT TENSION,
DROP SETS, 100s

EXERCISE	SETS[1]	REPS
Cable Incline Curl	3	6
Cable Incline Triceps Extension	3	6
Standing Cable Preacher Curl	3	8
Cable Kickback	3	8
Standing Cable Curl	3	12
Pushdown	3	12
Standing Calf Raise	1	100
Double Crunch	1	to failure

[1] After reaching initial failure on the last set of each exercise, reduce the weight by about 20% and continue repping to failure.

Workout No. 5
Whole Body

⟳ Looking to get a quick full-body burn? We've got just the thing. This 30-minute blast hits your entire body with a variety of movements, angles and equipment. The payoff is a head-to-toe workout that builds strength, burns fat and increases athleticism. Your muscles will beg for calories after this training session.

30-MINUTE METHODS: COMPOUND MOVEMENTS, VARIETY

EXERCISE	SETS	REPS
Dumbbell Deadlift to Step-Up[1] to Overhead Press	4	10
Lunge With Medicine-Ball Twist	3	16 steps
Medicine-Ball Swing	3	15 (each side)
Jump Squat	3	15
Speed Skater	3	to failure
Push-Up[2]	2	to failure

[1] alternate legs each rep

[2] Complete as many standard push-ups as you can. When you can no longer perform those, drop to your knees and rep to failure.

Bonus Tip
You can also use a dumbbell or kettlebell for this exercise

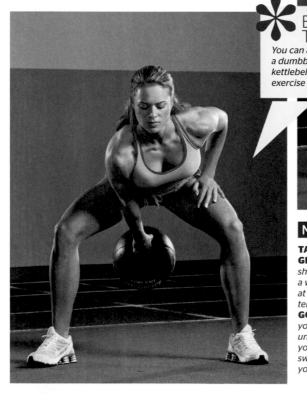

MEDICINE-BALL SWING

TARGET: *Whole body*
GET READY: *Stand with your feet wider than shoulder-width apart, then squat down to grasp a weighted ball between your feet. Lean forward at the hips about 45 degrees with your arm tensed, thighs just above parallel to the floor.*
GO: *Forcefully extend your hips and knees as you swing the ball forward and up in a wide arc until it's directly overhead. Immediately return to your starting squat position, letting the weight swing down along the same arc and between your legs. Repeat for reps, then switch sides.*

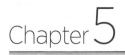

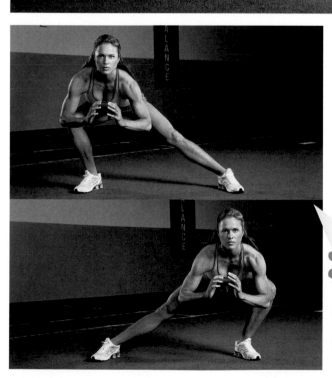

LUNGE WITH MEDICINE-BALL TWIST

TARGET: *Whole body*
GET READY: *Stand erect holding a light medicine ball in front of you, arms extended.*
GO: *Step forward with your right foot and descend into a lunge while simultaneously rotating your torso to the right, keeping your arms parallel to the floor. Don't let your knee pass your toes. Press through your right heel to lunge forward with your left foot while simultaneously rotating your torso to the left. Each step is one rep.*

SPEED SKATER

TARGETS: *Legs, glutes*
GET READY: *Stand with your feet wide apart, toes pointed out slightly. Descend into a squat until your thighs are roughly parallel to the floor, and bring your hands in front of your chest for balance.*
GO: *Lean to one side, allowing all of your weight to move over that knee as you extend and squeeze the opposite leg. After a brief count, lean to the other side and repeat.*

Extra Credit

Do this move slowly, squeezing both legs throughout. This is a great addition to any leg routine

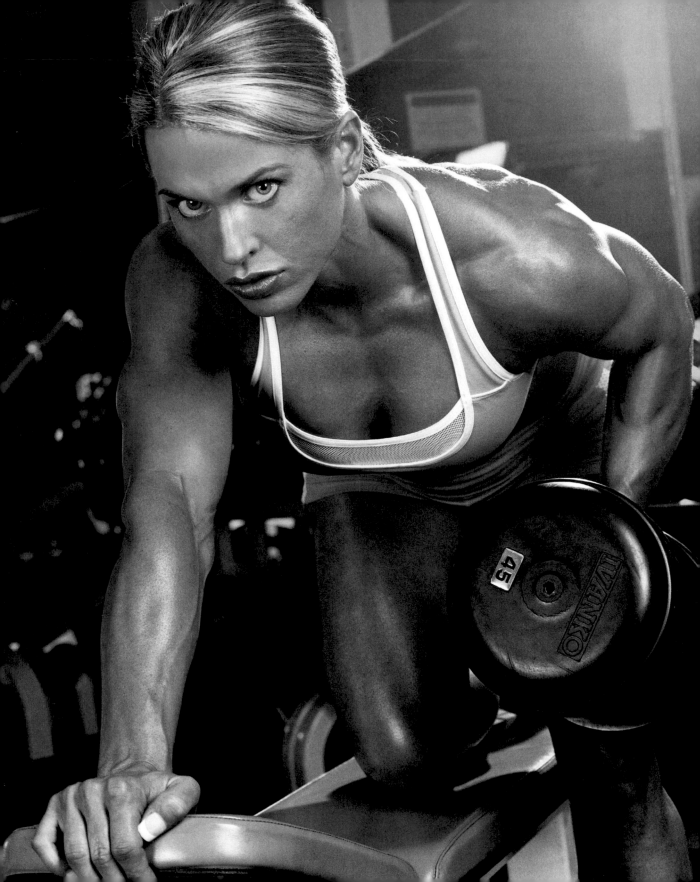

Chapter 6

Get Intense

Want to take your workouts to the next level? These four strength-building and fat-fighting intensity techniques will help you get there

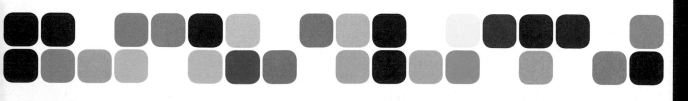

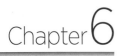

Chapter 6

It says so right on our cover: M&F HERS is a magazine for women who want more out of fitness and are willing to do what it takes to get it. Sometimes that means going well past the conventional boundaries that rigidly define the workouts — and physiques — of other women in the gym. But that's our readership.

Our readers know that one of the best ways to do that is to challenge your muscles, to demand more of your body and to expect compliance. Three sets of 12 simply won't do when it comes to sculpting the lean, glance-stealing physique you're after. With that in mind, we're laying down the training gauntlet. In keeping with our commitment to bring you more, we'll help you turn up the intensity with four proven advanced techniques for building the body you seek.

These techniques, though illustrated by a limited number of exercises here, can be broadly (yet sparingly) applied to your entire program. Whether a routine calls for drop sets, rest-pauses, supersets or negatives, you can use these intensity-boosters to build strength, burn more calories and turn your entire body into a well-defined metabolic machine. It won't take long for you to realize these techniques work; we're guessing that 24–48 hours after your first workout, you'll be reaching for your cell to schedule a rubdown with your masseuse.

You want more out of fitness, right? Well, just remember, you asked for it.

Drop Sets

With drop sets, you increase the intensity of a session by reducing the weight of an exercise and continuing to do reps. For example, if you can complete 12 reps of dumbbell rows, you'd immediately grab another dumbbell (one that's 20%–30% lighter) after your final rep and continue rowing, doing as many reps as possible before reaching for another lighter weight. This can be done numerous times. Regardless of how many drops you perform per set, it's considered one set. Keep the rest between drops minimal.

➲ **Benefit:** Drop sets help take your muscles beyond the limit of initial failure. Forcing them to continue contracting against lighter resistance will cause an elevated response of growth hormone and insulinlike growth factor-1, both of which are key for creating

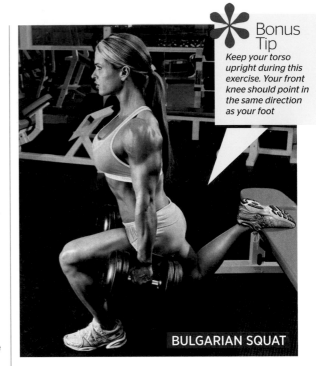

Bonus Tip
Keep your torso upright during this exercise. Your front knee should point in the same direction as your foot

BULGARIAN SQUAT

muscle, boosting strength and shedding bodyfat.

➲ **Use:** There are a couple of ways to incorporate drop sets. You can choose two exercises per muscle group, one compound and one isolation, and do three drop sets for each (see Chart 1A). Or you can make the last set of every exercise a drop set (see Chart 1B). As with any other intensity technique, it's important not to overuse drop sets. Limiting it to what's prescribed here is enough to help you push past plateaus.

Rest-Pause

The rest-pause technique helps boost your intensity by allowing you to tap into your creatine phosphate (CP) system. CP is responsible for supplying energy for powerful bursts, such as sprints and low-rep, explosive sets of weight training. CP lasts only briefly, but it's replenished during rest periods rather quickly. In other words, on a set of 6–7 reps done to failure, for example, your stores of CP that get you through the set are diminished fast. Once you begin to rest, your stores are almost fully replenished within 15–30 seconds. By using short rest periods within a set, then, you essentially prolong your CP levels and thus the set.

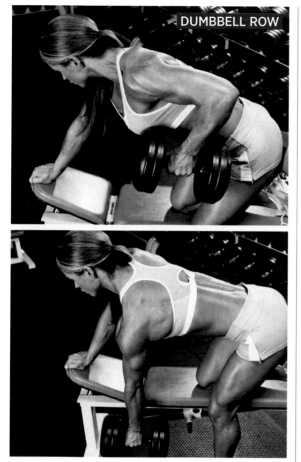

DUMBBELL ROW

Chart 1A

EXERCISE	SET	REPS	WEIGHT (LBS.)	REST
Dumbbell Row	1	12	40	—
		10	35	—
		8	25	2 min.
	2	11	40	—
		9	30	—
		7	25	2 min.
	3	9	30	—
		7	25	—
		4	20	—
Straight-Arm Pulldown	1	12	40	—
		10	35	—
		8	25	2 min.
	2	11	40	—
		9	30	—
		7	25	2 min.
	3	9	30	—
		7	25	—
		4	20	—

Chart 1B

EXERCISE	SETS	REPS
Barbell Row	4[1]	10
Wide-Grip Pulldown	3[1]	12
Seated Cable Row	3[1]	12

[1] On the final set, reduce the weight 20%–30% and continue repping to failure.

➲ **Benefit:** Rest-pause training allows you to take advantage of your explosive energy system, meaning you can complete extended, albeit interrupted, sets broken up by 15–20-second intervals. See Chart 2 for an example of how to use rest-pauses in the gym.

➲ **Use:** Try this type of training when strength is a priority. While some people train this way exclusively, we recommend you use it intermittently throughout your training cycles for a few weeks at a time, or simply cycle the bodypart with which you use it.

Supersets

Superset training puts two exercises back to back with no rest in between. It can be done for the same muscle group (a set of kickbacks followed by lying triceps extensions, for example) or for opposing bodyparts (that same triceps extension followed by a biceps curl). Superset workouts often have 2–3 exercise pairs for each muscle group.

➲ **Benefit:** The first and perhaps most obvious benefit of supersetting is time efficiency. Because you take limited rest between sets, these workouts are usually quicker than with other training methods. Second, if you superset opposing muscle groups, you'll actually be stronger on the second exercise (which is why you should vary which muscle you train first from workout to workout). Finally, supersetting's pace allows you to burn more total calories than straight-set training and standard rest periods.

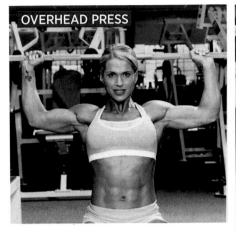

OVERHEAD PRESS

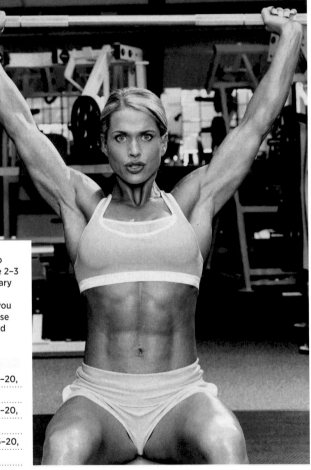

Chart 2

⮑ Select a weight that would cause you to fail at 5–7 reps but do only 2–3 reps, then stop. Rest for 15–20 seconds, then repeat the 2–3 reps. Continue this work/rest sequence as many times as necessary to reach your desired number of reps. Each set, then, comprises several small segments that make up a full rest-pause set. So if you do four small sets of 2–3 reps at a time, that makes one rest-pause set totaling 8–12 reps — and with a heavier weight than you could get 8–12 reps with in a straight, uninterrupted set.

EXERCISE	LOAD	SET	REPS/REST (SEC.)
Overhead Press	5RM	1	2/15–20, 2/15–20, 2/15–20, 2/15–20, 2/15–20
Upright Row	6RM	2	3/15–20, 3/15–20, 3/15–20, 3/15–20, 3/15–20
Lateral Raise	7RM	3	4/15–20, 4/15–20, 4/15–20, 4/15–20, 4/15–20

⮑ **Use:** Supersets are an ideal technique to use when your workout split pairs opposing muscle groups, such as quads and hamstrings (see Chart 3) or bi's and tri's, but they can enhance the intensity of any bodypart training. Perform an all-supersets routine for no more than 4–6 weeks to avoid becoming overtrained.

Negatives

Negative training involves further exhausting your muscles after you can no longer perform positive reps on your own. This is possible because your muscles are much stronger on the negative, or eccentric, portion of an exercise. Taking your muscles to negative failure increases the muscular damage, sparking further growth. But because it does cause a lot of damage, use this method infrequently — no more than every few weeks for a particular bodypart.

Ideally, you'll want to have a spotter help you through the positive portion of each rep. During the negative part of the move, you resist the weight on the way down and go as slowly as possible, aiming for about three seconds. If you can't resist the weight for at least three seconds, the set is over. At the bottom of the rep, your partner again assists you with the positive portion. Perform no more than 3–5 negatives after reaching positive failure.

If you don't have a partner, you can do certain

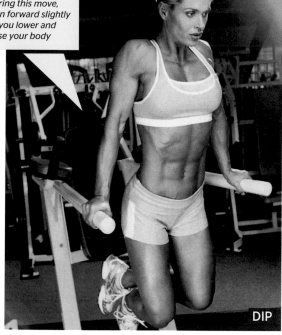

DIP

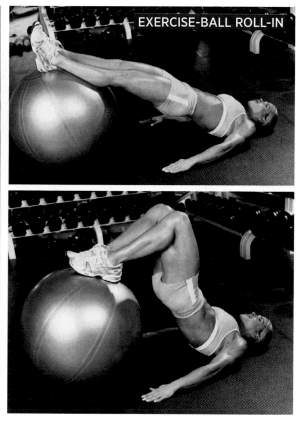

EXERCISE-BALL ROLL-IN

exercises unilaterally. Leg extensions, for example, can be done using your opposite leg to assist on the positive while the working leg resists the negative. On dumbbell preacher curls, you can use your nonworking arm to aid the working arm. Other self-spotting exercises include dumbbell front raises, dumbbell curls and overhead dumbbell extensions.

You can also use negatives on bodyweight exercises such as the dip. After you can no longer perform positive reps, use your legs to hop back up to the top position and then resist the downward path. Use the three-second rule here as well.

➔ **Benefit:** Negative training allows you to take advantage of when your muscles are strongest — on the eccentric, or negative, portion of the rep. Doing so after you've achieved positive failure causes further microtears in the muscle, making room for more muscle recovery and thus shapelier, stronger muscles.

➔ **Use:** Use negatives sparingly, ideally once every few weeks for a few exercises on a given bodypart. See Chart 4 for an example.

Chart 3

EXERCISE	SETS	REPS
Bulgarian Squat	3	10
— superset with —		
Reverse Lunge	3	10
Leg Extension	3	10
— superset with —		
Exercise-Ball Roll-In	3	10

Chart 4

EXERCISE	SETS	REPS
Bench Press	3[1]	10
Smith Machine Incline Press	3[1]	10
Pec-Deck Flye	3	10
Dip	3[1]	to failure

[1] Do negatives on the last set once you've reached positive failure. Select a weight that allows you to fail at the designated rep range.

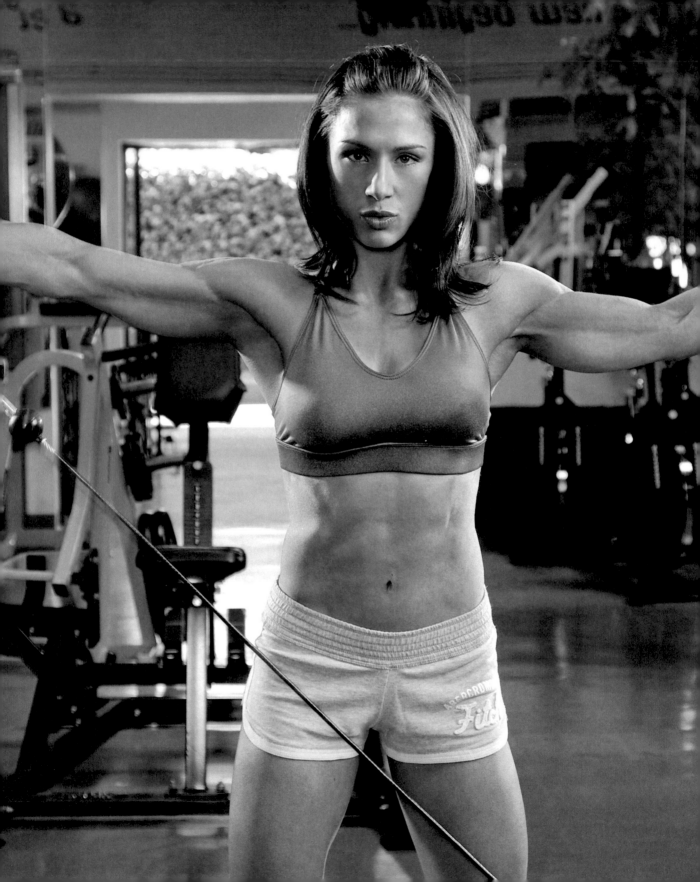

Smash HIT

Fewer sets, greater gains — that's the mantra behind high-intensity training, a workout philosophy designed to help you push your physique to new heights in less time

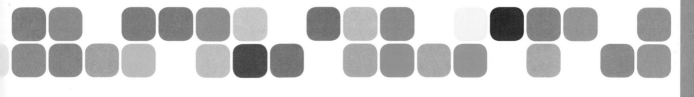

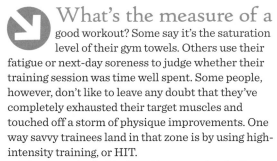

What's the measure of a good workout? Some say it's the saturation level of their gym towels. Others use their fatigue or next-day soreness to judge whether their training session was time well spent. Some people, however, don't like to leave any doubt that they've completely exhausted their target muscles and touched off a storm of physique improvements. One way savvy trainees land in that zone is by using high-intensity training, or HIT.

The reasoning behind HIT is pretty simple: Bombard each muscle group with one arduous set to failure or beyond to ensure that no fiber has gone untrained. It makes sense, too. If you perform multiple sets of an exercise, you cannot conceivably achieve maximum intensity on every working set (unless you're Super-woman). Consider HIT the shock-and-awe campaign of the workout world.

"In HIT, every working set must be taken beyond failure," says Jimmy Peña, MS, CSCS. "This requires the use of carefully selected and properly employed advanced training methods such as supersets, tri-sets and drop sets, all done with heavier-than-usual weight. Doing only one set per exercise allows a better chance of training with maximal intensity on every set."

This type of heart-pounding intensity may seem daunting, but it helps ensure you blast every muscle fiber you're working, which eventually leads to a tighter, shapelier appearance.

Training this way offers other perks, particularly for the time-crunched masses who love getting in and out of the gym quickly. Using a regular, high-volume day for legs as an example, you might perform five different exercises — squat, leg press, leg curl, leg extension and calf raise — for three sets each. That's 15 total sets. On a HIT leg day, you might do the same five exercises but with only one working set of each (not counting 1–2 warm-up sets of each move), or five sets total. The difference will be the intensity of each set.

"Your recovery time will be based on your own experience level and the bodypart worked," Peña says. "After a leg day, for example, you may need to stay away from training legs again for a week or more. For shoulders, maybe you can attack them again in 3–4 days."

The key to making HIT work for you, according to Peña, may lie in your mental resolve. "To train this way, you really have to be willing to go the extra mile."

Here, we present four distinct programs: One hits your upper body, one focuses on your lower body, one centers on shoulders and one targets arms.

Use the wide spectrum of exercises in these programs to gauge your body's reaction to HIT. From there, it's up to you how often you train this way, although we don't recommend doing so exclusively for more than a few weeks at a time. Find out for yourself why HIT is such a hit.

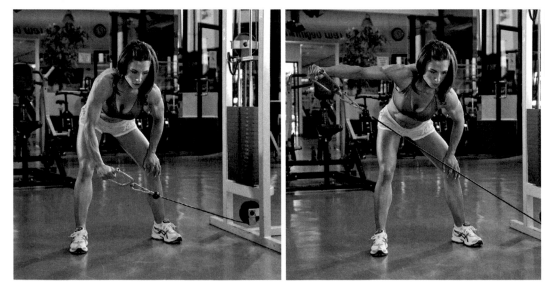

ONE-ARM BENT-OVER CABLE LATERAL RAISE

HIT Programs

USE THESE FOUR ROUTINES TO GET STRONG AND SHAPE UP IN A HURRY

The nature of HIT precludes you from working out like this every day, but that's part of the benefit — higher intensity means your body will need more time to recover but will come back stronger. Each of these programs includes a precise frequency recommendation. Of course, if you've never trained this way before, you may want to experiment with only one of these programs per week — within the framework of your current routine — until you become accustomed to HIT's unique demands.

No. 1 Upper-Body Cable Crush

This constant-tension, cable-based program forces you to work one side of your body at a time, taxing your core muscles. Go through the entire sequence of exercises in circuit fashion twice as a warm-up, completing 10 reps (not to failure) each time. Move through the entire cycle of exercises using one side of your body before repeating with the other side. Each exercise puts your body at a greater mechanical advantage so you get stronger with every move, even though you're fatiguing.

Frequency: Since this is a comprehensive upper-body program, you shouldn't do it more than twice a week, allowing 3–4 days of rest between sessions. In between, train your abs and lower body and perform your usual schedule of cardio.

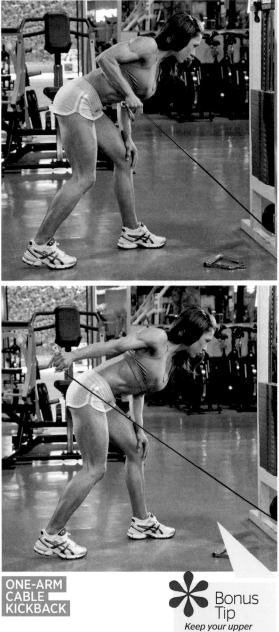

ONE-ARM CABLE KICKBACK

EXERCISE	SETS[1]	REPS[2]
One-Arm Bent-Over Cable Lateral Raise	1	4,6,8,10,12,20
One-Arm Cable Kickback	1	4,6,8,10,12,20
One-Arm Standing Low-Cable Row	1	4,6,8,10,12,20
One-Arm Cable Lateral Raise	1	4,6,8,10,12,20
One-Arm Cable Curl	1	4,6,8,10,12,20
One-Arm Cable Overhead Press	1	4,6,8,10,12,20
One-Arm Cable Crossover	1	4,6,8,10,12,20

[1] doesn't include two lighter warm-up sets of 10 reps

[2] Start with a weight you can barely handle for four reps and then repeatedly drop the load by 20%–30%, or 1–2 plates on the weight stack. The subsequent rep targets are suggestions. If you more than double your number of reps each time, you've dropped too much. Each drop in the sequence should be done to complete muscle failure, for five total drops.

✷ **Bonus Tip**
Keep your upper arm at your side. Don't lift your elbow to raise the weight; that takes emphasis off your triceps

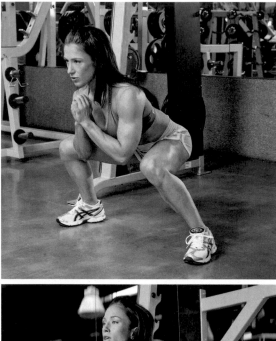

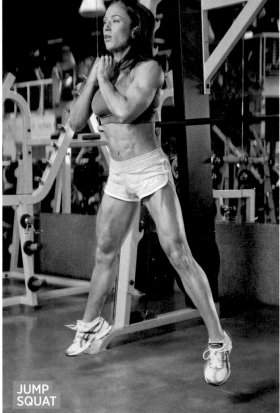

JUMP SQUAT

No. 2 Lower-Body Blast

You'll notice that this lower-body routine is conspicuously devoid of single-joint exercises such as the leg extension and leg curl. Instead, we attack your entire lower-body musculature with compound moves to up the intensity factor. You'll complete one working set of each move — after a full-body warm-up and two passes through each exercise with lighter weight — and finish with a final, grueling set of 30 on the Smith machine squat. Might we suggest a hearty postworkout stretching session?

Frequency: This routine targets a trouble area for many women, but that doesn't give you license to do it every day. The explosive nature of several of these exercises requires you to be completely rested to perform at optimal levels. Aim to do this routine twice — and no more than three times — a week, allowing 24–48 hours of recovery between bouts.

EXERCISE	SETS[1]	REPS[2]
Smith Machine Squat	1	4,6,8,10,12,20
Jump Squat	1	4,6,8,10,12,20
Sissy Squat	1	4,6,8,10,12,20
Romanian Deadlift	1	4,6,8,10,12,20
Smith Machine Squat	1	30

[1] Doesn't include two lighter warm-up sets of 10 reps

[2] Start with a weight you can barely handle for four reps and then repeatedly drop the load by 20%–30%. The subsequent rep targets are suggestions. If you more than double your number of reps each time, you've dropped too much. Each drop in the sequence should be done to complete muscle failure, for five total drops.

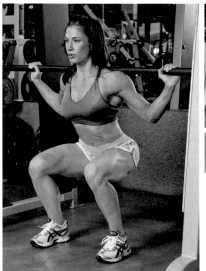

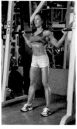

SMITH MACHINE SQUAT

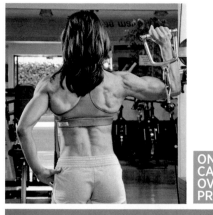

ONE-ARM
CABLE
OVERHEAD
PRESS

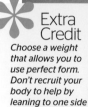

Extra Credit

Choose a weight that allows you to use perfect form. Don't recruit your body to help by leaning to one side

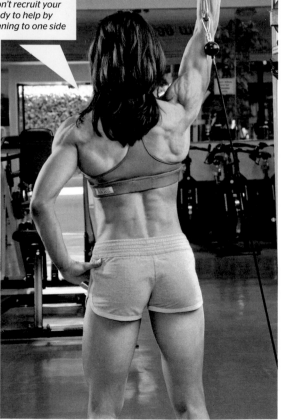

No. 3 Shoulder Smash

The use of lighter weight on this tri-set will have your shoulders begging for mercy in no time flat. Although you use a comfortable weight — roughly your 10-rep max — this varied-angle approach engages the three heads of your deltoids differently each time. The emphasis, as you'll quickly find, is on your front delts, but your middle and rear delts are called into play heavily as your front delts fatigue. Again, we recommend a sufficient full-body warm-up, followed by at least two lighter sets of each exercise listed.

Frequency: Although we have some recommendations in mind, we're certain you'll realize after the first session that doing this routine more than once a week could be tough. If shoulders are an area of concern for you, you can try it a second time, but only after 3–4 full days of rest with no shoulder work in between. Remember, your shoulders are comprised of several small muscles, so beware of overtraining them.

EXERCISE	SETS[1]	REPS
Barbell Front Raise	1	1
Upright Row	1	1
Overhead Press	1	1

[1] Perform these exercises as a one-rep tri-set. Select a weight you can handle for 10 reps on the front raise, then perform one rep of each exercise. Repeat this sequence until you reach complete muscle failure on the front raise. Then do only the upright row and the overhead press in sequence until you fail on the upright row. At that point, continue doing only overhead presses until you reach failure on that move.

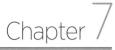

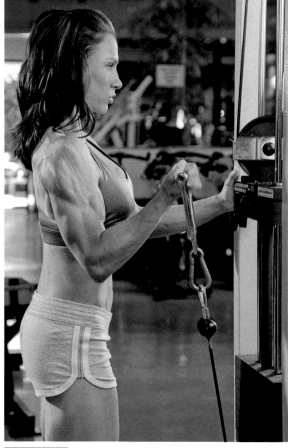

ONE-ARM CABLE CURL

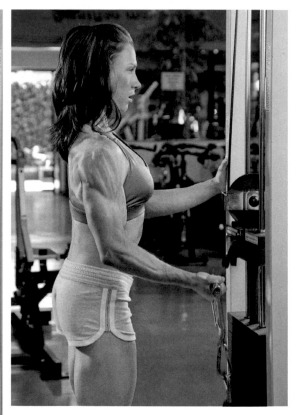

No. 4 Fire Arms

This superset-based HIT program for arms will definitely have your bi's and tri's burning. Again, the idea is to go to complete muscle failure on one exercise — in this case, you're basically doing drop sets for biceps and triceps, only in superset fashion.

Frequency: Everyone wants to have a great set of arms, and this routine delivers. Although it's made up of only two exercises, its intensity level is off the charts. Complete this program once or twice per week, getting at least 3–4 days of rest between sessions.

EXERCISE	SETS	REPS[1]
Standing Cable Curl	1	6,10,15,6 to failure
— superset with —		
Cable Overhead Extension		

[1] After two light warm-up sets of 10 reps on each exercise, perform a heavy set of six on cable curls, then immediately do a set of six on cable overhead extensions. Without rest, decrease the weight slightly and hit a set of 10 for each. Again without rest, decrease the weight and do a set of 15 for each. Then go back to the starting weight and do as many reps as possible, aiming for six reps to failure.

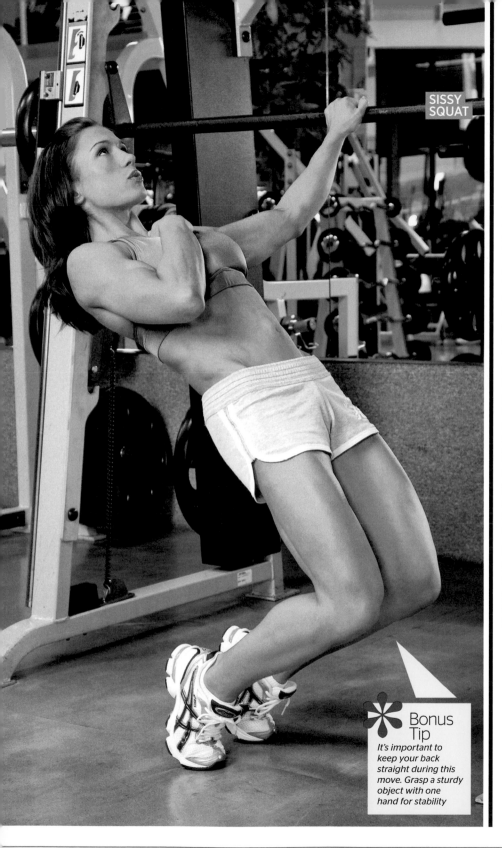

SISSY
SQUAT

Getting Intense

Here are some broad strokes on the techniques you'll employ in these HIT programs

➲ **DROP SETS:** After completing your reps in a heavy set, quickly strip an equal amount of weight from each side of the bar, select lighter dumbbells or adjust the pin on the weight stack. Continue to do reps until you fail, then strip off more weight to complete even more reps.

➲ **SUPERSETS:** Perform two exercises for the same or different muscle groups back to back with no rest in between.

➲ **TRI-SETS:** Perform three consecutive exercises for one muscle group in nonstop sequence. Rest after the third exercise.

✱ Bonus Tip

It's important to keep your back straight during this move. Grasp a sturdy object with one hand for stability

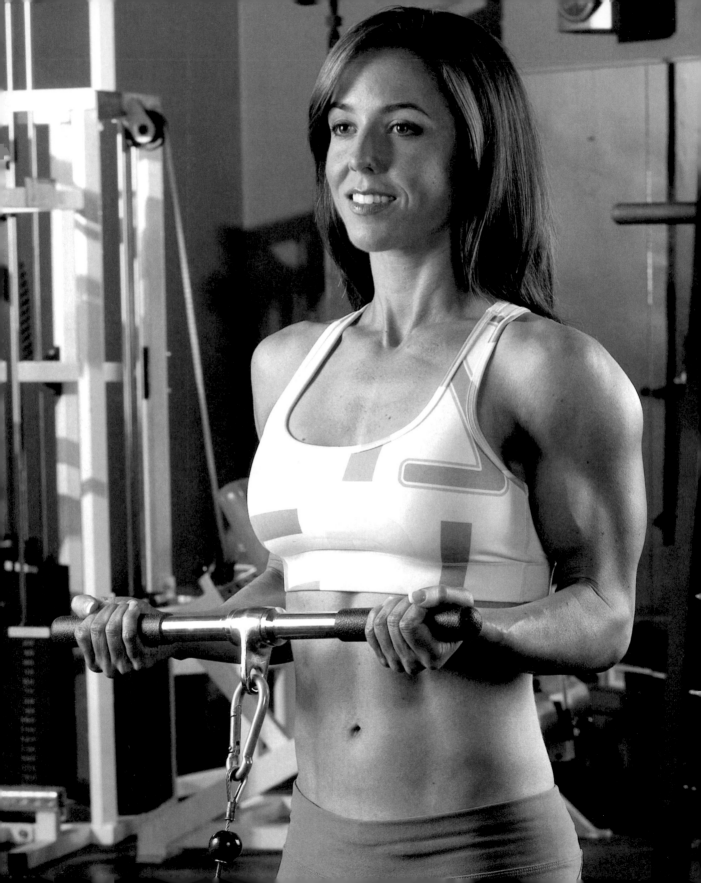

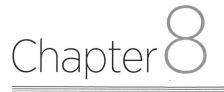

Three x Seven

We re-engineer the classic 21s format into a muscle-sculpting, full-body workout

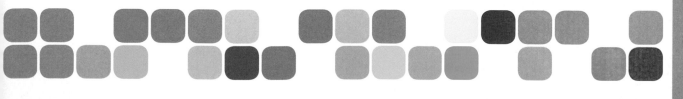

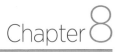

The fitness world is full of workout techniques that float in and out of vogue depending on the trade winds of trend. One effective high-intensity method that's often forgotten is 21s. Generally done with biceps curls, 21s involves doing seven reps through the bottom half of the range of motion (ROM), seven reps through the top half and seven complete reps, with no rest in between.

The benefits are legion since different portions of the ROM target different muscle fibers, further emphasizing each bodypart. Moreover, you get an intensity boost that can help push your lean muscle development to the next level.

Although this technique has been practiced for decades, we offer a new and improved take. We've moved the full-ROM reps from the end of the set to the beginning, then have you immediately do seven reps through the bottom half of the ROM followed by seven reps through the top half to complete 21 reps. Choose a weight that's 50%–70% of your 10-rep max.

Our version is more beneficial for several reasons. Working through the full ROM first acts as a warm-up. That way when you do the bottom half of the move, where the muscle is weakest, you have more strength. And in the final reps when fatigue sets in, you'll utilize the ROM in which the muscle is strongest. The last seven reps will still be challenging, however, as the muscle is fatigued from the previous 14 reps.

Making this routine even more unique is how we applied 21s to each bodypart. For this approach to truly be effective, you must focus on single-joint or isolation movements such as biceps curls, pushdowns, lateral raises, flyes, leg curls and leg extensions. This allows you to target a single muscle group; multijoint exercises, on the other hand, involve numerous bodyparts for overall mass and strength gains.

Our program is a full-body training split done three times a week. Try performing the 21s workout on Monday and Friday and the standard multijoint workout in between. This way you train the majority of fibers in each major muscle group with both isolation and multijoint moves each week.

For best results, follow this program for 4–6 weeks. If a full 21s program doesn't fit into your schedule, you can do this workout as a one-time substitute when you want to switch things up or you're short on time. Either way, the routine provides your muscles with variety, which will help advance your progress in the gym.

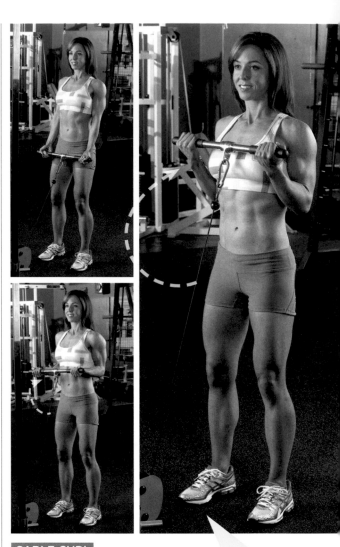

CABLE CURL

TARGET: *Biceps*
GET READY: *Stand erect with your feet shoulder-width apart and grasp a straight bar attached to a low-pulley cable using a shoulder-width grip.*
GO: *Perform the first seven reps through the full range of motion. For the next seven, start at full-arm extension and stop when your elbows are just shy of 90-degree angles. Finish by starting with your forearms just below parallel to the floor and curling all the way up. Keep your elbows fixed at your sides throughout.*

Bonus Tip
To keep constant tension on the cable, make sure you're standing far enough away from the machine

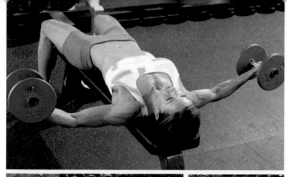

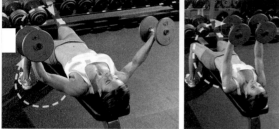

DUMBBELL FLYE

TARGET: *Chest*
GET READY: *Lie faceup on a flat bench grasping a dumbbell in each hand, extend your arms straight out to your sides and bend your elbows slightly.*
GO: *Do seven full-range-of-motion reps, bringing the weights together over your chest. For the next seven, start with your hands in line with your shoulders and lift the weights until your arms form 45-degree angles to the floor. Finish by starting with your arms at the 45-degree position and stopping when your hands meet above your chest.*

Workouts 1+3 (21s)

EXERCISE	SETS/REPS	REST
CHEST		
Dumbbell Flye	4/21	1–2 min.
SHOULDERS		
Lateral Raise	4/21	1–2 min.
BACK		
Straight-Arm Lat Pulldown	4/21	1–2 min.
TRICEPS		
Pushdown	4/21	1–2 min.
BICEPS		
Cable Curl	4/21	1–2 min.
QUADS		
Leg Extension	4/21	1–2 min.
HAMSTRINGS		
Leg Curl	4/21	1–2 min.
ABS		
Sit-Up	4/21	1 min.

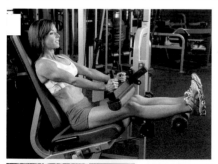

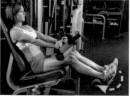

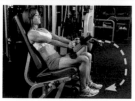

LEG CURL

TARGET: *Hamstrings*
GET READY: *Sit in the machine so your knees line up with the axis of rotation. Start with your legs near full extension.*
GO: *Do seven reps through the full range of motion, forcefully contracting your hamstrings. Perform the next seven by starting at full extension and stopping just shy of your knees forming 45-degree angles. Do the last seven reps with your knees starting just short of the 45-degree position and going to full contraction.*

Workout 2 (Standard multijoint)

EXERCISE	SETS/REPS	REST
QUADS		
Squat	4/8–10	1–2 min.
HAMSTRINGS/GLUTES		
Romanian Deadlift	4/8–10	1–2 min.
CHEST		
Incline Press	4/8–10	1–2 min.
BACK		
Barbell Row	4/8–10	1–2 min.
SHOULDERS		
Overhead Press	4/8–10	1–2 min.
BICEPS		
EZ-Bar Curl	4/8–10	1–2 min.
TRICEPS		
Close-Grip Bench Press	4/8–10	1–2 min.
CALVES		
Standing Calf Raise	4/10–15	1 min.
ABS		
Hanging Leg Raise	4/to failure	1 min.

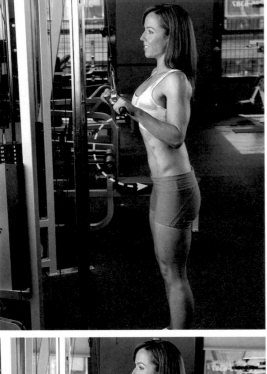

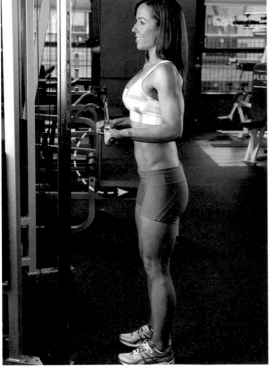

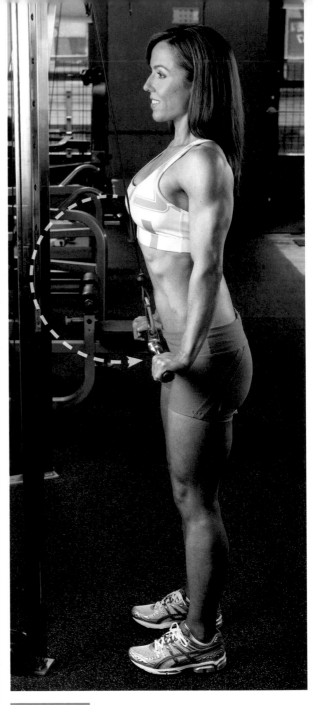

PUSHDOWN

TARGET: *Triceps*
GET READY: *Stand erect grasping a straight bar attached to the upper-pulley cable with your elbows pinned to your sides, forearms just above parallel to the floor.*
GO: *Do seven reps pushing the bar to full-arm extension and squeezing your tri's at the bottom. Perform another seven reps starting at the same point and stopping when your forearms form 45-degree angles to your body. For the final seven, start at the 45-degree position and stop when your arms are fully extended.*

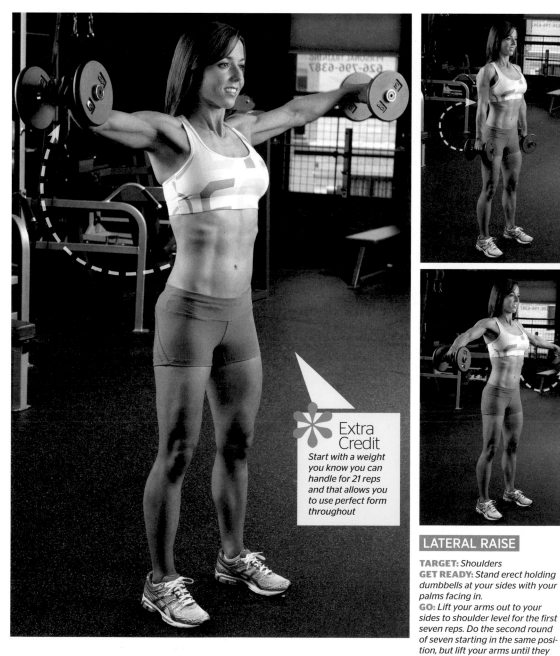

Extra Credit

Start with a weight you know you can handle for 21 reps and that allows you to use perfect form throughout

LATERAL RAISE

TARGET: *Shoulders*

GET READY: *Stand erect holding dumbbells at your sides with your palms facing in.*

GO: *Lift your arms out to your sides to shoulder level for the first seven reps. Do the second round of seven starting in the same position, but lift your arms until they form 45-degree angles to your torso. For the final seven reps, start with your arms at the 45-degree position and stop when they come parallel to the floor.*

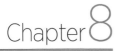

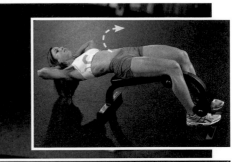

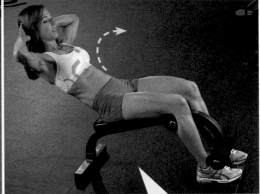

Bonus Tip

As your abs grow stronger, consider boosting the intensity by holding a weight plate across your chest

SIT-UP

TARGET: *Abs*
GET READY: *Use an ab bench and anchor your feet under the rollers.*
GO: *With a flat back, curl your torso toward your knees for seven reps. For the next group of seven, curl up until your torso is at a 45-degree angle to the floor. Finish by starting at the 45-degree position and stopping when your torso is perpendicular to the floor.*

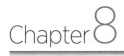

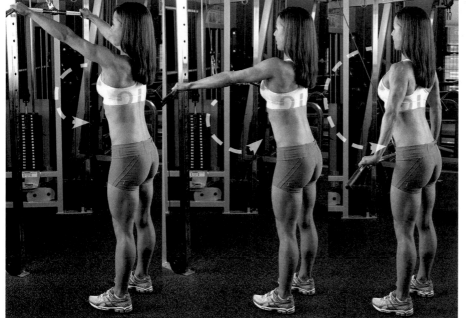

STRAIGHT-ARM LAT PULLDOWN

TARGET: *Back*
GET READY: *Grasp a lat pulldown bar attached to a high-pulley cable using a wide, overhand grip. Start with the weight a few inches off the stack.*
GO: *Do seven reps through the full range of motion, pulling the bar to your thighs. For the next seven, start at the same point but stop when your arms form 45-degree angles to your torso. To finish, start with your arms at the 45-degree position and stop when the bar touches your thighs.*

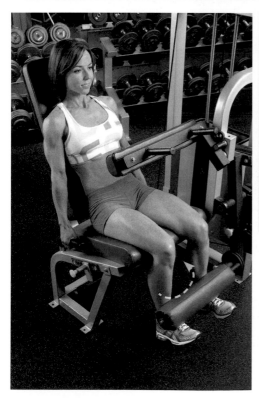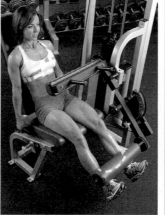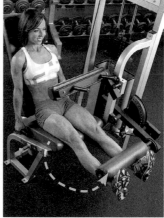

LEG EXTENSION

TARGET: *Quads*
GET READY: *Sit in the machine so your knees line up with the axis of rotation. Start with your knees bent just less than 90 degrees.*
GO: *Use a full range of motion for seven reps, squeezing your quads at the top. Perform seven more reps by starting at the 90-degree position and stopping just past where your knees form 45-degree angles. For your final seven, begin with your knees just shy of the 45-degree position and go to full extension.*

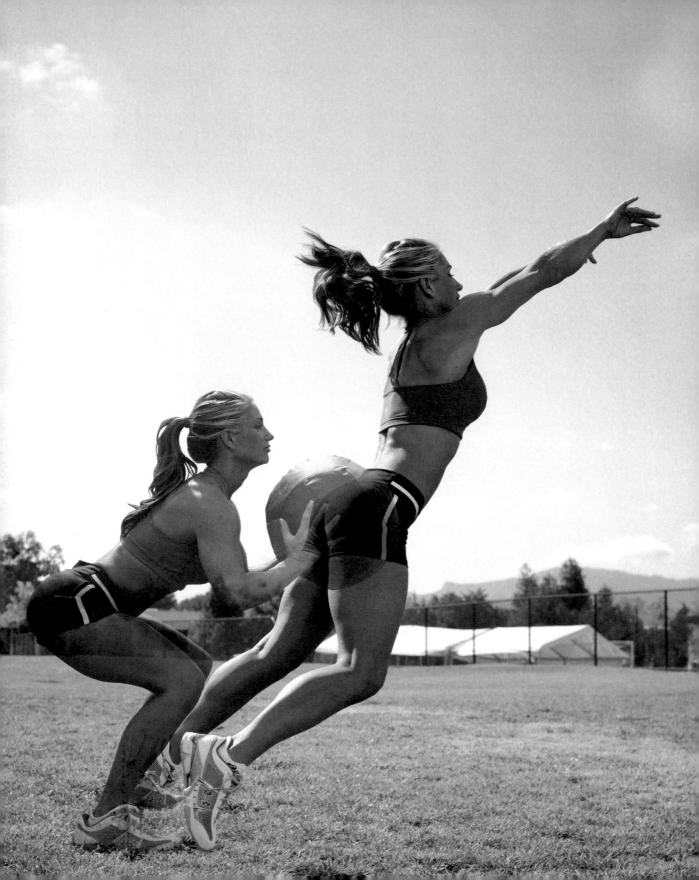

Throw, Jump, Lunge

Get out and play as you reshape your physique with this challenging medicine-ball circuit

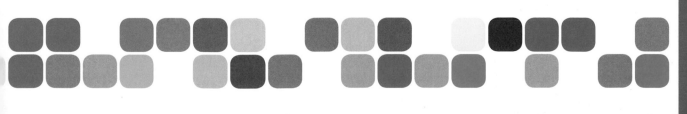

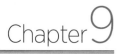 **Chances are pretty good** that you've held a medicine ball. You may have even used one while lunging, squatting or twisting. But the chances are equally good that you've never realized the full potential of a med ball and you're skeptical of just how well these weighted spheres can produce real-world results.

If you've never trained in the great outdoors with one, then your skepticism is warranted. Because that's where these affordable, low-maintenance weights offer you the ability to perform a vast number of exercise combinations to burn fat, build strength and inject much-needed variety into your routine.

"I use medicine-ball throws with all my clients," says Rachel Rose, former elite rower and New York personal trainer. "I've found that women love to get outside and do something less conventional than typical machine circuits and treadmill or elliptical work."

The real advantage to taking these old-school tools outside is in the dynamic possibilities they offer. When you lift weights in the gym, the environment limits the speed and force with which you can move a free weight or machine handle. To generate maximum force on the bench press, for example, you'd need to throw the barbell or dumbbells into the air. But hurling weights across the gym is fraught with all kinds of legal and physical implications.

Medicine balls taken outside, on the other hand, can be thrown with all the force you can muster, which means there's no limit to how much speed or effort you use. Simply put, you can train without constraint and from every conceivable angle. Athletes run, jump and throw with freedom of movement, and that's the most effective way to train with medicine balls.

In fact, this focus on movement as opposed to isolated bodyparts can help give you that sleek, athletic look. This routine will teach you to move more fluidly, recruit more motor units and use your entire body to complete a task, and it'll raise your heart rate using high-intensity interval training (HIIT), commonly regarded as the best way to burn fat.

"Athletes look great because they train athletically," Rose says. "This sounds obvious, but it's not because most people don't know how athletes train. Medicine balls are a staple for elite athletes, and they're so versatile that any woman can incorporate them into her training program."

Medicine-Ball Circuit Training

This workout offers a comprehensive sampling of what's possible with medicine-ball training. You'll start with the throw and chase, a super full-body warm-up that can be used for any sport. After that, you'll go through a series of HIIT-style movements designed to burn fat, build explosive power and work various energy systems to get you in better overall shape. These moves are most effective when performed at the start of a session because your central nervous system is relatively untaxed, and you can move the ball faster and more forcefully. Finally, you'll perform three strength-building exercises: the overhead walking lunge, and medicine-ball push-up and push crunch.

EXERCISE	SETS	REPS	REST
Throw and Chase	2	100 yards	1 min.
Half-Squat Jump Throw and Chase	1	10	1 min.
Half-Squat Jump-Bounce Throw and Chase	1	10	1 min.
Backward Overhead Throw and Chase	1	10	1 min.
Side-Twist Throw and Chase	1	10	1 min.
Kneeling Coil Throw	1	10	1 min.
Overhead Walking Lunge	2	20 steps	1 min.
Medicine-Ball Push-Up	2	10	1 min.
Medicine-Ball Push Crunch	2	20	30 sec.

THROW & CHASE
(Not Shown)

TARGET: *Whole body*
GET READY: *Begin at one end of a grass or artificial-turf field holding a medicine ball with both hands at chest level.*
GO: *Throw the ball one of a variety of ways — chest pass, twisting throw, backward overhead throw — then chase it. When you reach the ball, pick it up and throw it another way in the same direction.*

HALF-SQUAT JUMP THROW & CHASE
(Not Shown)

TARGETS: *Quads, hips, glutes*
GET READY: *Stand with your feet shoulder-width apart and knees bent. Hold a medicine ball at chest level with your palms facing your torso slightly.*
GO: *Descend into a half-squat, then jump forward and throw the ball as far as you can using a two-hand chest pass. Use your forward momentum to chase the ball, then pick it up and repeat.*

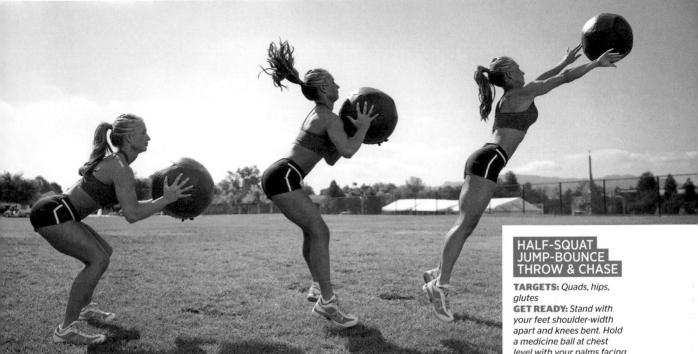

HALF-SQUAT JUMP-BOUNCE THROW & CHASE

TARGETS: *Quads, hips, glutes*

GET READY: *Stand with your feet shoulder-width apart and knees bent. Hold a medicine ball at chest level with your palms facing your torso slightly.*

GO: *Descend into a half-squat and jump as far forward as you can. When you land, immediately jump again as far as you can, simultaneously launching the ball as far as you can using a two-hand chest pass. Keep your contact with the ground as short as possible between jumps. Use your forward momentum to chase the ball, then pick it up and repeat.*

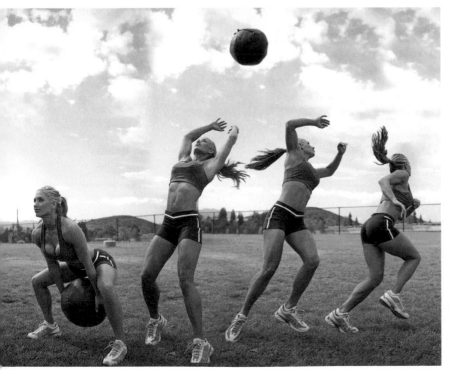

BACKWARD OVERHEAD THROW & CHASE

TARGETS: *Hamstrings, lower back*

GET READY: *With your feet slightly wider than shoulder width, squat down and hold a medicine ball with both hands between your legs.*

GO: *Extend your knees, hips and arms, and throw the ball as high and as far behind you as you can. Turn and chase it, pick it up and repeat.*

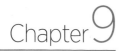

Chapter 9

SIDE-TWIST THROW & CHASE

TARGETS: *Quads, hips, obliques*
GET READY: *Stand erect with your feet slightly wider than shoulder width and your toes pointed forward. Hold a medicine ball at chest level, arms extended.*
GO: *Twist as far to one side as you can, then toss the ball as far as you can to the opposite side as you rotate that direction. Chase the ball, then pick it up and repeat to the opposite side. Make sure you propel the ball using your torso, not your arms or hands.*

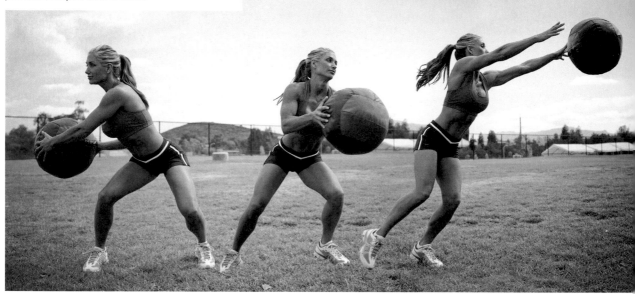

MEDICINE-BALL PUSH CRUNCH

TARGET: *Abs*
GET READY: *Lie faceup with your knees bent about 90 degrees and your feet flat on the ground. Hold a medicine ball with both hands, arms extended directly over your face.*
GO: *Keeping the ball above you, contract your abs to raise your upper body off the ground. Hold for a second, then return to the start position.*

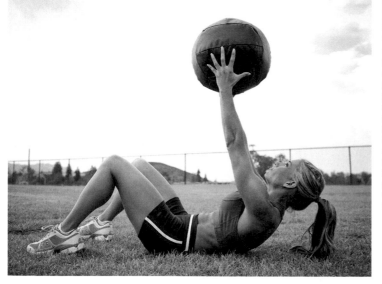

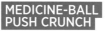

OVERHEAD WALKING LUNGE

TARGETS: *Quads, glutes, shoulders*
GET READY: *Stand erect with your feet shoulder-width apart holding a medicine ball in front of you with both hands.*
GO: *Raise the ball overhead and step forward into a lunge. Descend until your front knee forms a 90-degree angle and your back knee nearly touches the ground. Lower the ball to waist level and drive through your front foot to bring your back leg forward and return to standing. Repeat using the opposite leg.*

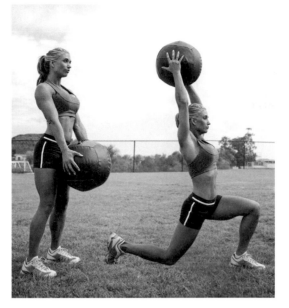

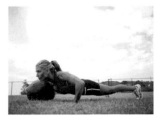

MEDICINE-BALL PUSH-UP

TARGETS: *Chest, triceps*
GET READY: *Get in push-up position with a medicine ball nearby.*
GO: *Place one hand on the ball and one on the ground, and perform a push-up. Reverse your hand position and repeat, alternating hands for reps.*

KNEELING COIL THROW

TARGETS: *Hamstrings, chest, triceps*
GET READY: *Kneel on the ground holding a medicine ball at chest level with your palms facing your torso slightly.*
GO: *Using a two-hand chest pass, throw the ball as far as you can and land in a push-up position. Retrieve the ball and repeat. If you perform this movement against a wall, push off the wall back to a kneeling position, retrieve the ball and repeat. If you work with a partner, have her roll the ball back to you.*

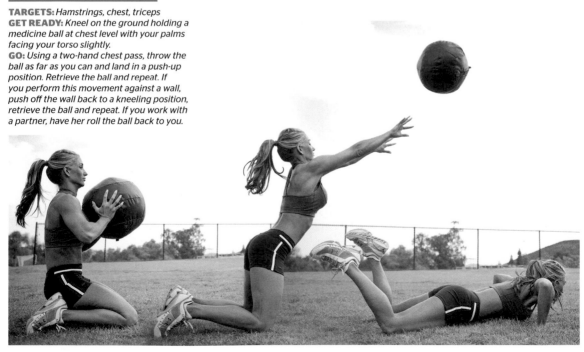

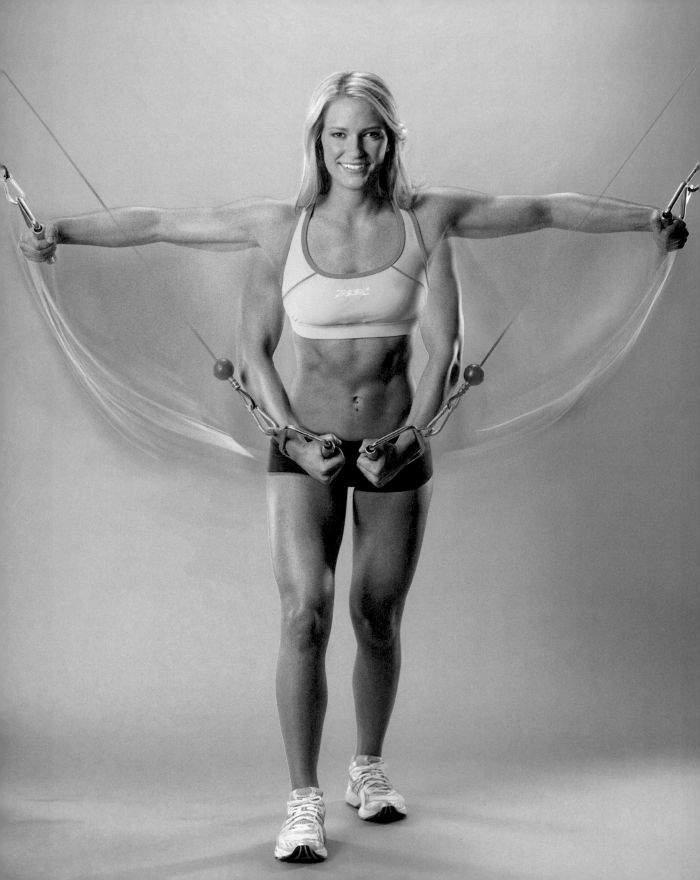

Be a Super Woman

Doing supersets in superfast style is the best way to burn fat and get lean. Here's how to superset effectively for optimal results

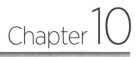 Talk about your all-time great training discoveries. Whoever first tried the squat (known way back when as a deep knee bend) uncovered the single best exercise for sculpting the legs and glutes. Likewise, the creators of the push-up and crunch were resourceful enough to find moves that could be performed when they didn't have time to go to the gym. Brilliant!

Then there's the superset, arguably the single greatest training technique this side of full-range-of-motion reps and progressive overload. (To refresh your memory, a superset involves doing two exercises back to back with no rest in between.) When Joe Weider perfected this gem, he found a way to effectively intensify a workout and burn more calories, all while saving precious time in the gym.

We think so much of training with supersets that we not only incorporate them into programs addressing any number of goals but we're also more than happy to design workouts consisting of nothing but supersets, which is exactly what you'll find here. And when you do your supersets in rapid-fire fashion, you're on the road to achieving a leaner, more sculpted physique super-quick.

Sets With Benefits

Supersetting isn't simply a means of speeding up your workout. That's a bonus, sure, but doing exercises back to back produces many desirable responses in the body that can lead to a leaner, shapelier physique. Here are a few:

➔ **Supersets increase growth-hormone (GH) levels.** This is an important factor. Women, by nature, don't have nearly as much testosterone as men do. For the sake of looking feminine, this is a good thing, but at the same time it's one reason women carry less muscle and more bodyfat than men. That said, females rely much more on GH for muscle recovery and growth than men do, which is key to getting leaner. In fact, after weight workouts GH levels rise much higher in females than in men. When you eliminate rest periods, as you do when supersetting, GH levels rise even more than when you perform straight sets. Moreover, increasing GH results in a marked increase in lipolysis, the release of fat from fat cells, which allows the fat to travel to the muscles to be burned as fuel. This process is vital when you want to shed bodyfat.

Superset Samples

➔ These six superset routines utilize three different training splits: a two-day split, where you complete each workout twice a week; a three-day split, where you perform each workout 1–2 times a week; and a full-body workout (which includes two different tri-sets) to be done 2–3 times a week.

TWO-DAY SPLIT
DAYS 1 & 3: UPPER BODY

EXERCISE	SETS	REPS
CHEST/BACK		
Cable Crossover	4	10
— superset with —		
Seated Cable Row	4	10
BACK/SHOULDERS		
Lat Pulldown	4	10
— superset with —		
Dumbbell Overhead Press	4	10
BICEPS/TRICEPS		
EZ-Bar Preacher Curl	3	12
— superset with —		
Pushdown	3	12

Alternate which exercise you perform first in each superset every other workout.

DAYS 2 & 4: LOWER BODY + ABS

EXERCISE	SETS	REPS
LEGS		
Leg Extension	4	10
— superset with —		
Dumbbell Lunge	4	10
Lying Leg Curl	4	15
— superset with —		
Smith Machine Squat	4	15
ABS/LOW BACK		
Crunch	4	20
— superset with —		
Back Extension	4	20

Alternate which exercise you perform first in each superset every other workout.

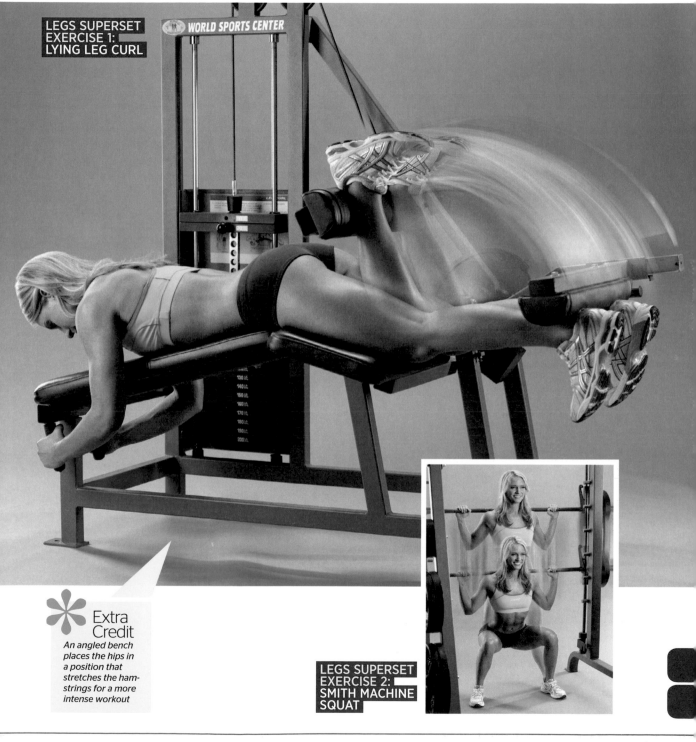

LEGS SUPERSET EXERCISE 1: LYING LEG CURL

WORLD SPORTS CENTER

Extra Credit
An angled bench places the hips in a position that stretches the hamstrings for a more intense workout

LEGS SUPERSET EXERCISE 2: SMITH MACHINE SQUAT

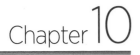

Chapter 10

➔ **Supersetting burns more calories.** Typically, when you superset exercises, you do roughly twice as much work in the same amount of time as when you perform straight sets, since you do your second exercise when you'd otherwise be resting. This is beneficial for obvious reasons, namely because losing weight comes down to burning more calories than you take in. And burning more calories means increasing your metabolism.

➔ **Supersetting makes you stronger.** Studies show that when you superset opposing muscle groups (for example, chest and back or biceps and triceps), you'll be stronger on the second exercise. For example, if you do dumbbell presses for chest followed by seated rows for back, you'll be stronger than usual on the rows. This helps not only those seeking to get stronger but also anyone looking to get leaner and tighter. The stronger you are on a given exercise, the more weight you can use and/or the more reps you can do, which in turn burns more calories and builds more muscle, both of which increase metabolism.

Perfect Pairs

Supersets come in many different forms, and a wide variety of exercise pairings have proven effective. As we noted, training opposing muscle groups together is common — for instance, chest and back, bi's and tri's, abs and lower back, quads and hamstrings. This involves doing two opposing movements back to back which, in addition to the aforementioned benefits, promotes muscular balance. If you always follow a chest exercise with a back exercise (or vice versa), for example, you minimize the chance that one muscle group will overpower the other.

Another common method is to superset exercises for a single bodypart: lunges with hack squats, pushdowns with lying triceps extensions, hanging leg raises with crunches and so on. This increases intensity and focus on one muscle group, typically as a means of bringing up a lagging area. For example, if your shoulders are a weakness, you could superset overhead presses with upright rows or lateral raises with bent-over raises.

Superset pairings don't need to be so systematic, however. If you'd prefer to superset a chest exercise with abs, or an upper-body exercise with a lower-body movement, go right ahead. All such combinations will

Three-Day Split
DAY 1: CHEST + BACK + SHOULDERS

EXERCISE	SETS	REPS
CHEST		
Dumbbell Bench Press	3	12
— superset with —		
Dumbbell Flye	3	12
BACK		
Seated Cable Row	4	12
— superset with —		
Straight-Arm Lat Pulldown	4	12
SHOULDERS		
Upright Row	3	12
— superset with —		
Lateral Raise	3	12

DAY 2: LOWER BODY

EXERCISE	SETS	REPS
LEGS		
Leg Press	3	12
— superset with —		
Leg Extension	3	12
Seated Leg Curl	3	15
— superset with —		
Romanian Deadlift	3	15
CALVES		
Standing Calf Raise	3	20
— superset with —		
Seated Calf Raise	3	20

DAY 3: TRICEPS + BICEPS + ABS

EXERCISE	SETS	REPS
TRICEPS		
Lying Triceps Extension	3	12
— superset with —		
Dumbbell Overhead Extension	3	12
BICEPS		
Alternating Dumbbell Curl	3	12
— superset with —		
Cable Curl	3	12
ABS		
Hanging Leg Raise	3	15
— superset with —		
Machine Crunch	3	15

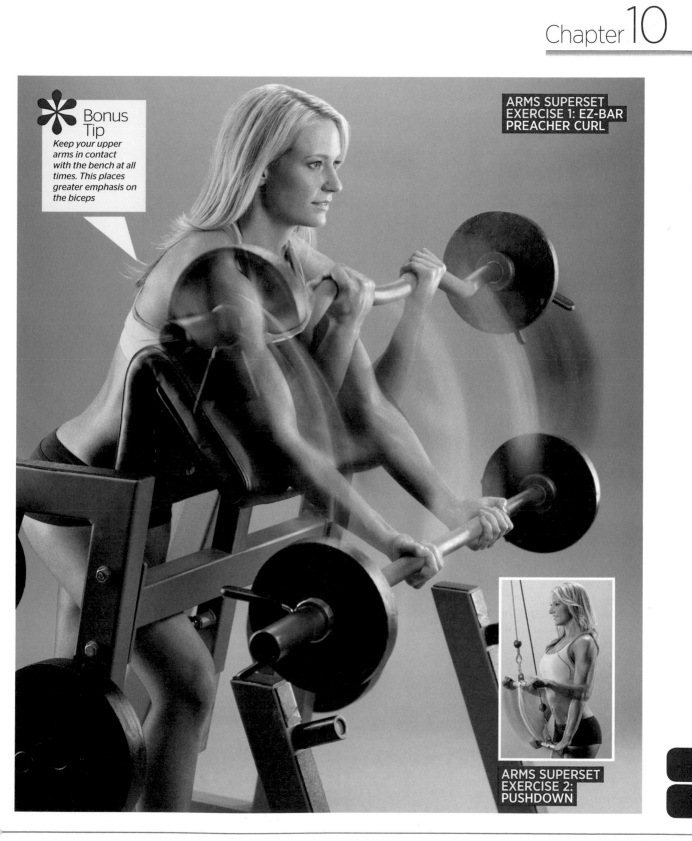

Bonus Tip

Keep your upper arms in contact with the bench at all times. This places greater emphasis on the biceps

ARMS SUPERSET EXERCISE 1: EZ-BAR PREACHER CURL

ARMS SUPERSET EXERCISE 2: PUSHDOWN

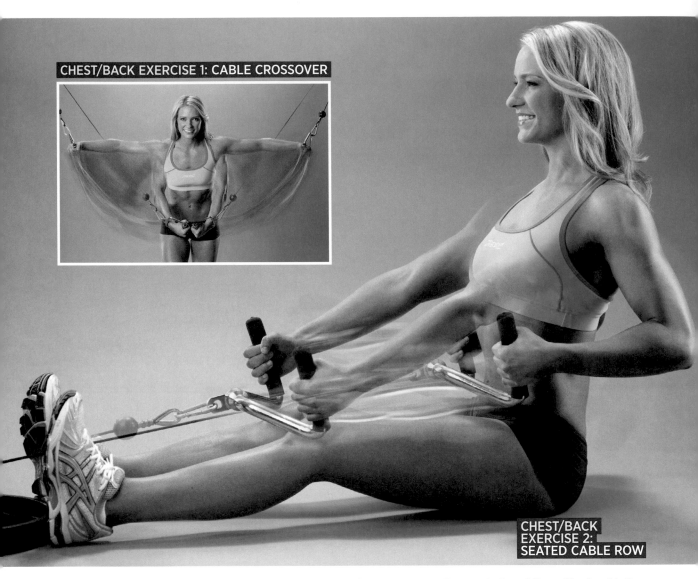

CHEST/BACK EXERCISE 1: CABLE CROSSOVER

CHEST/BACK EXERCISE 2: SEATED CABLE ROW

help increase the efficiency of your workouts while maximizing calorie-burning via shortened rest periods. Nor are you required to stick to supersets of only two exercises; advanced trainees can combine three exercises (called tri-sets) or more (giant sets) to burn even more calories and keep the heart rate elevated that much longer. Tri-sets and giant sets, like supersets, can include exercises for the same or opposing muscle groups. For example, you can do a giant set for back that consists of pull-ups followed by barbell rows, lat pulldowns and seated cable rows, or a tri-set

that consists of lunges for legs followed by dumbbell presses for chest and cable curls for biceps.

The sample workouts are made up entirely of supersets — no straight sets. We include a variety of supersetting methods, from opposing muscle group pairings to supersets for the same bodypart. Incorporate all of them into your training or even devise your own pairings. You'll find our routines to be fast-paced and intense, and they'll hit more muscle in less time. What more could you ask for of one training technique?

Super Guidelines

1) **To build the speed factor into your supersets,** rest only as long as it takes you to move from one exercise to the next. Theoretically, you're not resting between exercises, but in reality a few seconds will elapse between the end of one set and the start of the next. The key is to minimize that time.

2) **Between supersets, rest longer.** If you never rest during the workout, you won't be able to lift as much weight, which can actually decrease the amount of work you do. To maintain adequate strength levels, rest 1–2 minutes between each superset.

3) **Typically, you do multijoint exercises first in a superset.** If your superset includes a compound exercise (for example, dumbbell bench presses) and an isolation exercise (say, flyes), do the compound move first, which will allow you to use maximum weight. Doing the isolation movement first is called pre-exhaustion — a worthy technique, but one that's more advanced.

4) **Swap the order of exercises.** Especially when supersetting opposing muscles, alternate which exercise you perform first. For example, in a biceps/triceps superset, don't always do biceps first (or vice versa). Switch it up every other superset pairing, or every other workout, to promote balanced muscle growth.

5) **You may need to go lighter.** Because supersets are typically more intense than a straight-sets routine, be prepared to use slightly lighter weight, especially late in the workout when you're fatigued and when supersetting exercises for the same bodypart. For example, if you superset barbell and dumbbell curls, chances are you'll need to go lighter than normal on the dumbbell version.

6) **Choose two-arm exercises.** If you do an arms superset that consists of barbell curls and dumbbell kickbacks, you'd generally do one arm first on the kickbacks and then switch sides. This means the first arm gets no rest and the second arm gets a decent amount after doing curls, so

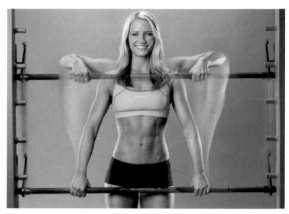

Full-Body Split
TO BE DONE ON NONCONSECUTIVE DAYS

EXERCISE	SETS	REPS
CHEST/SHOULDERS/TRICEPS		
Tri-set:		
Incline Press	3	10
Dumbbell Overhead Press	3	12
Pushdown	3	15
BACK/BICEPS		
T-Bar Row	3	10
— superset with —		
Dumbbell Incline Curl	3	15
LEGS		
Tri-set:		
Leg Press	3	12
Lying Leg Curl	3	15
Standing Calf Raise	3	20
ABS/LOW BACK		
Crunch	3	25
— superset with —		
Back Extension	3	15

you'll likely be stronger on the second arm, causing a potential imbalance. To avoid this, stick to two-arm exercises when supersetting. (Of course, you can do kickbacks with both arms, which also solves the problem.) Another solution is to superset one-arm exercises such as dumbbell concentration curls and kickbacks: Either do one set of each exercise with one arm, then switch sides; or train one arm and then the other on curls before moving on to kickbacks.

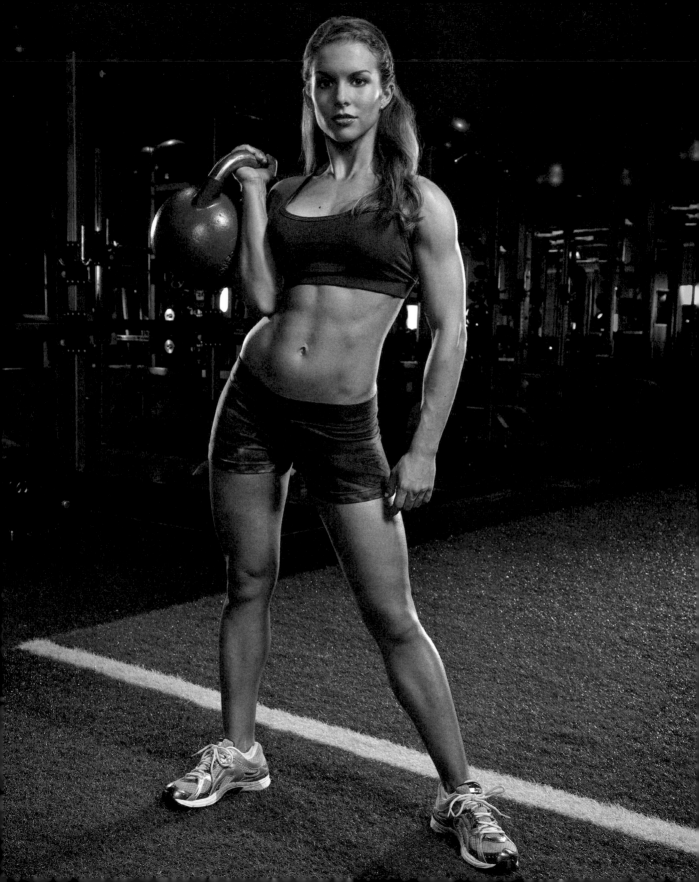

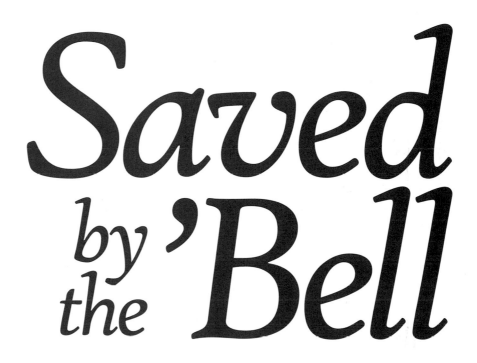

Chapter 11

Saved by the 'Bell

Here's a comprehensive introduction to the kettlebell, America's hottest new workout tool

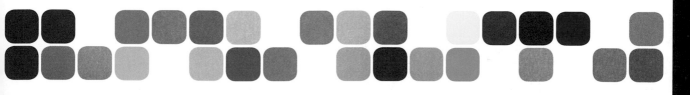

There's a long list of reasons for women to start swinging a kettlebell, the medieval-looking cannonball with a handle that has been popping up in more and more gyms. It's a time-saving three-in-one workout tool that delivers cardio, strength and flexibility benefits.

It's also a space-saving, inexpensive ($20–$70) "gym in your hand" that provides enough variety to keep you busy for 30 minutes. It's a superb total-body conditioner that blasts your core, builds coordination and balance, and even helps you recover from injuries. It develops power through natural movements that are tough to achieve with machines. You can do it in your living room or backyard, or at the beach or park. Anyone can do most of the exercises — even the technical ones — on the first day, yet they leave you worked and winded.

But perhaps its most standout feature is right behind you: "You get awesome glutes," says Alysia Gadson, a certified kettlebell instructor, personal trainer and spinal-care specialist in Newport Beach, California. "It not only looks awesome but it works."

That's a big deal because most glutes don't work, says Andrea DuCane, the world's first female master kettlebell trainer. "Our society suffers from 'gluteal amnesia' — when the glute muscles lose their ability to fire," she explains. "All the sitting we do, plus quad-centric activities such as cycling and long-distance running, trains them to stay flaccid. That means our hip flexors and lumbar muscles must do all the work in keeping us upright, leading to a host of back and flexibility problems."

Pavel Tsatsouline brought a pair of developed glutes with him to the U.S. in the late 1990s. The thoroughly ripped former Soviet special-forces trainer also brought the kettlebells he used to build them. He didn't think anyone would be interested in the devices, which had been a mainstay of strength workouts in Russia and Scandinavia for 200 years.

Thanks in part to Tsatsouline, kettlebells are now popular with men and women, DuCane is a master RKC (Russian Kettlebell Challenge) trainer

and kettlebells are one of America's hottest new workout phenomena, popping up in commercial gyms and jamming sporting-goods store shelves.

For a safe, effective, challenging introduction to kettlebells, M&F HERS consulted with the experts to formulate this eight-exercise super-sequence that works you from head to toe. Designed for maximum safety, variety and motivation, the progression starts with the basics: the deadlift squat, swing and turkish get-up. Then it ramps up to the clean, press, windmill and high pull, and finally to the peak of the Olympic lifts — the body-blasting snatch — leaving you with serious bragging rights and an exhilarating sense of achievement.

The Program

Lauren Brooks, a personal trainer in Encinitas, California, was so happy with her kettlebell results a couple of years ago that she largely quit using conventional weight machines. "I don't really need them anymore. Kettlebells are a better workout," says Brooks, a level 2 RKC instructor. To enhance safety, she starts all her clients with an 18-pound kettlebell and gradually increases the weight. (Very strong women use 35-pounders; elite lifters use 50–60-pounders.) She recommends doing 3–5 30-minute workouts per week.

Those 30 minutes shouldn't begin with the iconic, butt-blasting swing, says Brooks, and most kettlebell instructors agree. Instead, this plan warms you up with the deadlift squat, a controlled, nonballistic exercise that most instructors recommend for its ability to correct your biomechanics.

For most exercises, do three sets of 10–15 reps, resting 30 seconds between each set. Perform fewer reps for the turkish get-up (four reps per set, two per side) and windmill (2–3 reps per side). Do exercises 1–3 on Day 1 and the remaining moves on Day 2. Combine Days 1 and 2 into an über-workout when you really want to test yourself.

Whatever mix of exercises you do as your fitness improves over time, don't push the workout beyond 30 minutes. "It's risky to go too long," DuCane says. "Kettlebells work the stabilizing muscles the whole time and they fatigue, too, which can be dangerous."

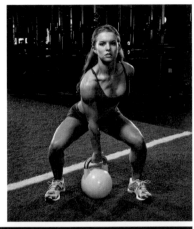

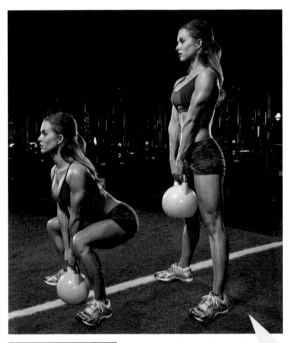

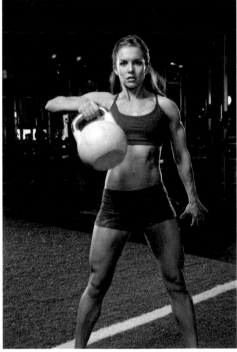

DEADLIFT SQUAT

TARGETS: *Legs, glutes*
GET READY: *Stand erect with your feet wider than shoulder width, toes pointed out slightly. Squat down and grasp a kettlebell in front of you with both hands, arms extended.*
GO: *With your back flat, return to standing by straightening your legs and squeezing your glutes, keeping the weight close to your body. Push your hips forward at the top of the move.*

Bonus Tip

As with the regular squat, make sure your knees don't go past your toes. Descend as if to sit in a chair

CLEAN

TARGETS: *Legs, glutes, back, shoulders*
GET READY: *Stand erect with your feet shoulder-width apart. Squat down and grasp a kettlebell between your legs with one hand.*
GO: *Pull the weight straight up as you extend your knees and hips. As the weight reaches waist level, rotate your shoulder and bring your elbow underneath so the kettlebell is racked at chin level. It should rest against your forearm, your arm tight against your rib cage. Repeat for reps, then switch sides.*

The Routine

EXERCISE	SETS	REPS	REST
DAY 1			
Deadlift Squat	3	10–15	30 sec.
Swing	3	10–15	30 sec.
Turkish Get-Up	3	2	30 sec.
DAY 2			
Clean	3	10–15	30 sec.
Press	3	10–15	30 sec.
Windmill	3	2–3	30 sec.
High Pull	3	10–15	30 sec.
Snatch	3	10–15	30 sec.

NOTE: For safety, limit your workout time to 30 minutes.

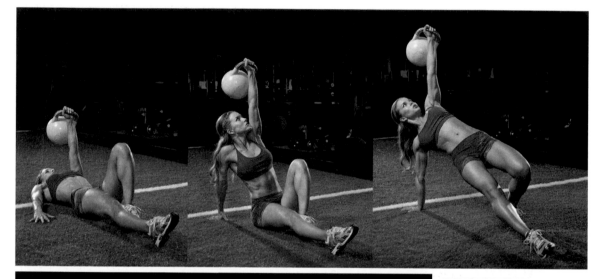

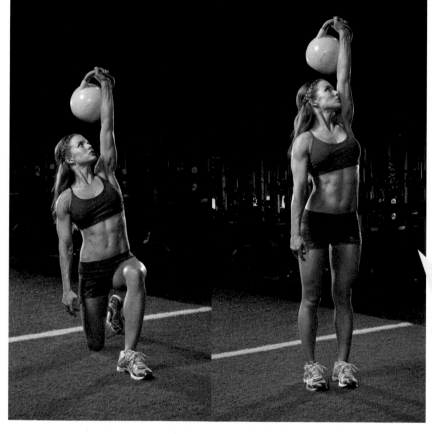

TURKISH GET-UP

TARGETS: *Legs, glutes, back, shoulders*

GET READY: *Lie faceup on the floor and hold a kettlebell in your left hand directly above your shoulder. Keep your elbow locked, wrist straight and your eyes on the weight.*

GO: *Bend your left knee so your foot is flat on the floor, sit up and tilt your hips so you're supported on both feet and your right hand. Swing your right leg under your body and prop yourself up on that knee. Press through your right knee and left foot to stand upright. Reverse the movement to lie back down. The kettlebell remains elevated throughout. Perform only two reps per side, per set.*

✳ Extra Credit

Like the deadlift, the Turkish get-up will work your entire body when done properly. Do just two reps per side, per set

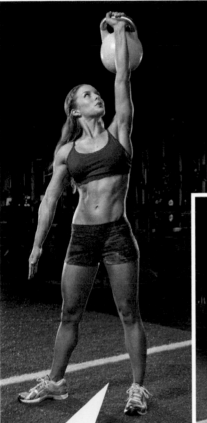

WINDMILL

TARGETS: *Shoulders, abs*
GET READY: *Stand erect with your feet shoulder-width apart and hold a kettlebell overhead with your left hand, keeping your eyes on the weight.*
GO: *Slowly lean sideways at the hips as you keep your arm vertical. Touch your right hand to the floor with your arm 90 degrees to your torso. Perform only 2-3 reps per side, per set.*

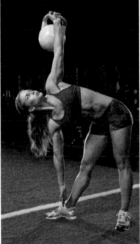

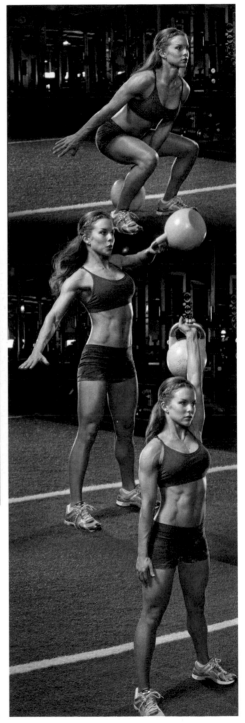

✳ Bonus Tip

Turn the foot you reach toward to a 45-degree angle. Always focus on the weight and keep your back flat

SNATCH

TARGETS: *Legs, glutes, back, shoulders*
GET READY: *Stand erect with your feet shoulder-width apart. Keeping your back flat, squat down and grasp a kettlebell between your feet with one hand.*
GO: *Pull the weight off the floor by extending your knees and hips, keeping it close to your legs. As it reaches knee level, shrug and swing the weight into a high pull. Without pausing, bend your elbow and push your hand through the handle. Press the kettlebell overhead and lock out your elbow at the top. Repeat for reps, then switch sides.*

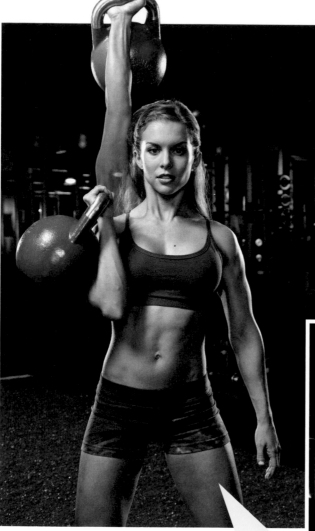

HIGH PULL

TARGETS: *Legs, glutes, back, shoulders*
GET READY: *Stand erect with your feet shoulder-width apart. Squat down and grasp a kettlebell between your feet with one hand.*
GO: *Arch your back and position your shoulders over the weight. Pull it off the floor by extending your knees and hips, keeping your arm straight. When the weight reaches knee level, explosively shrug your shoulders and pull the kettlebell to shoulder level, with your elbow above and to the outside of the weight. Lower under control. Repeat for reps, then switch sides.*

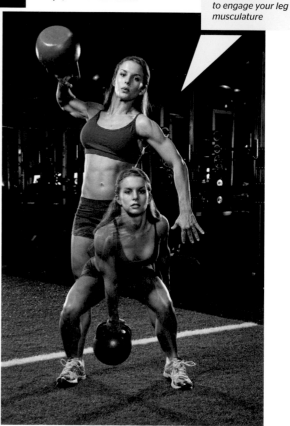

✻ Bonus Tip
To increase the momentum of the weight, push through your heels to engage your leg musculature

PRESS

TARGET: *Shoulders*
GET READY: *Begin with the kettlebell racked at chin level.*
GO: *Press the weight powerfully overhead, rotating your wrist so your palm faces forward. Lock your elbow, keeping your biceps next to your ear. Repeat for reps, then switch sides. Once you've mastered the clean and the press separately, you can combine them into one exercise.*

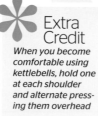

✻ Extra Credit
When you become comfortable using kettlebells, hold one at each shoulder and alternate pressing them overhead

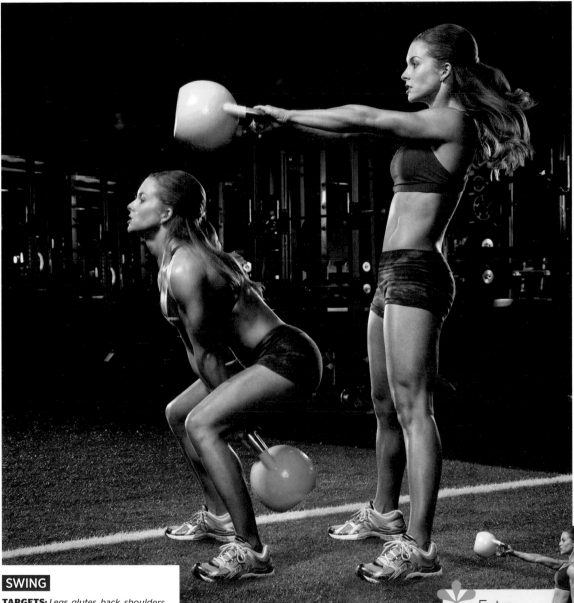

SWING

TARGETS: *Legs, glutes, back, shoulders*
GET READY: *With your back flat, squat down and grasp a kettlebell between your legs with both hands.*
GO: *Extend your knees and hips, and use the momentum to swing the weight in an arc to chest level, arms extended. Keep your shoulders down and back; don't let them round or track forward. Allow gravity to return the kettlebell to the start as you bend your knees and hips.*

✳ Extra Credit

Do one-arm swings and hand-to-hand swings, in which you toss the weight from one hand to the other at the top of the movement

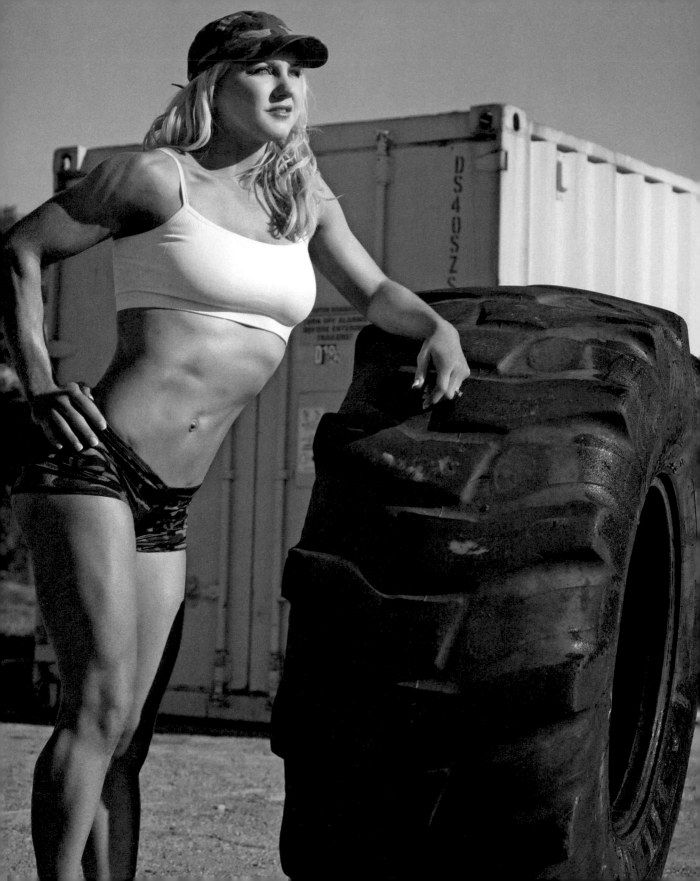

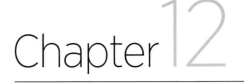

Chapter 12

Beyond 300

The Hollywood-born workout that took the fitness world by storm is no longer just for guys

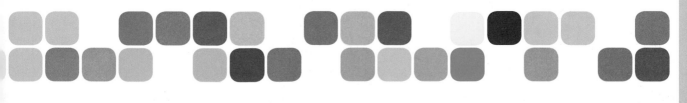

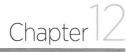
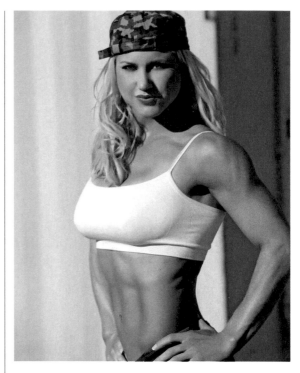

Four years after 300 hit the big screen, it's clear that the film's furthest-reaching contributions will have nothing to do with special effects or mangled Greek history. Instead, the movie will be remembered for inspiring a training sensation dedicated to emulating the actors' well-oiled physiques. Soon after the film was released, gyms all over the country began offering *300*-inspired workouts designed to cut fat while building muscle, strength and endurance.

The downside? The workouts were grueling, overwhelming beginners and intermediates alike. And despite their unorthodox structure, the routines were fairly inflexible in terms of weight and exercises. For most women, looking at the Spartans is quite different from looking *like* the Spartans (the beards might be tough to pull off, anyway).

"The 300 workouts were made for men," IFBB fitness pro Julie Lohre says. "I can't control the same weight a man can, and the last thing I want to do when I'm working out is get hurt. It's important to push yourself but also remain safe."

Like many, Julie was bored with countless gym hours spent in 8–10-rep, station-after-station drudgery. "I wanted something different that still trained the whole body," she says. So she came up with a solution. Pulling from her vast experience as a top fitness competitor, she created a program specifically for women that can take them "Beyond 300."

"It's fun and challenging to do something new, and there's a lot of pride in being able to say you completed this workout," Julie says. "It's so much fun to get down and dirty, and do a variety of exercises while [racing] against the clock. This workout is like being a kid on a playground."

This Is...Kentucky

Creating her own workout program is nothing new for Julie, who placed eighth in the 2007 Fitness Olympia. She has been forging her own path since she began competing in 2003.

A gymnast and cheerleader as a youth, Julie fell into corporate lethargy after college. "I went from being active in college to sitting at a desk every day for five years," Julie says. "Once I had my son, I really wanted to get back in shape. Every woman wants to feel

good about her body and have energy."

Julie wasted no time. Five months to the day after giving birth, she entered and won her first contest, which qualified her for others. "I was still breastfeeding backstage," she says. "For my first three competitions, I was still nursing."

Now Julie teaches scores of women who compete in fitness, and most love the Beyond 300 workout. "The two things everyone notices most are increases in strength and endurance. To be able to do 50 box jumps and 50 push-ups is an accomplishment. Plus, it benefits the entire body."

If you're new to the gym, Beyond 300 can appear daunting. Even if you have a good base of strength and endurance, this workout can be hard, and you'll ache all over the next day. The upside — besides a break from your stale routine — is it offers a great way to measure your personal fitness. By charting the weight you use, and especially the time it takes you to complete the workout, you can easily track your progress.

"If you aren't sure [how much] weight to use, just go through each exercise one at a time and don't worry about the clock," Julie says.

Beyond 300

EXERCISE	REPS
Wide-Grip Assisted Pull-Up	25
One-Arm Clean and Press	25 (each side)
Box Jump	50
Lying Leg Raise With Dumbbells	50
Romanian Deadlift	50
Elevated Push-Up	50
Wide-Grip Assisted Pull-Up	25

1) Pacing

The workout is timed and the number of reps is fixed, so the faster you perform this routine, the higher your level of fitness. Julie's record is 22:39, but most of her students take more than 30 minutes to finish their first time through. Regardless of where you start, racing the clock is an objective way to measure progress.

2) Rest

Beyond 300 is designed to be performed with minimal rest: "Rest only as much as you absolutely have to," Julie says. You can rest between reps but not between exercises; finish one exercise and then hustle to the next.

3) Level

Even though this workout was devised for advanced female athletes, a few basic modifications can make it suitable for almost anyone. Simply use a weight you feel comfortable with and break down the exercises into manageable chunks. You might do 20 reps, catch your breath, then finish the set by doing "subsets" of 5–10 reps at a time.

4) Frequency

Julie recommends doing this workout once a week for eight weeks in addition to your normal training split.

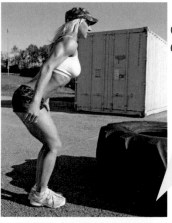

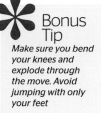

❊ Bonus Tip

Make sure you bend your knees and explode through the move. Avoid jumping with only your feet

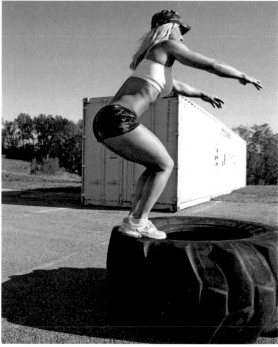

BOX JUMP

TARGET: *Quads*
GET READY: *Stand erect with your feet hip-width apart facing a 20-inch-high box (or step or bench).*
GO: *Squat down slightly, then push through your quads to jump onto the box with both feet. Return to the start position as quickly as possible. If you're worried your vertical jump won't be high enough, start out with an aerobic step and gradually increase the height by adding risers.*

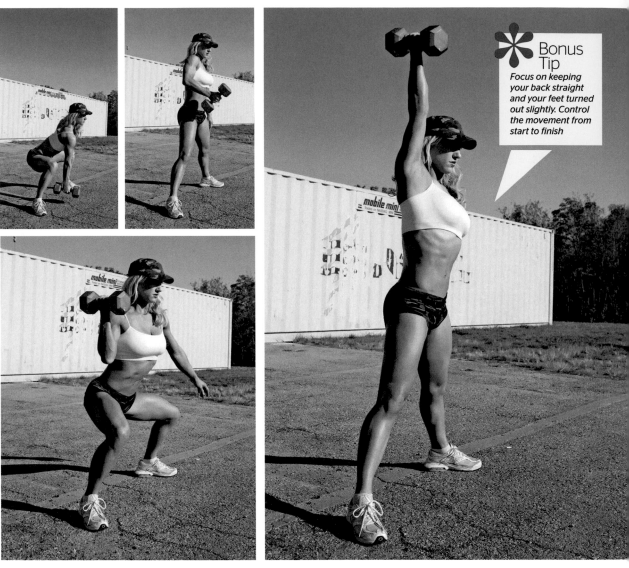

Bonus Tip

Focus on keeping your back straight and your feet turned out slightly. Control the movement from start to finish

ONE-ARM CLEAN AND PRESS

TARGETS: *Legs, glutes, back, shoulders*
GET READY: *Stand with your feet just wider than shoulder-width apart and hold a dumbbell between your legs with one hand. Keep your chest lifted and torso facing forward.*
GO: *Descend into a squat without letting your knees move past your toes, then explode upward, smoothly cleaning the weight to your shoulder and dipping underneath it. Press the dumbbell overhead as you return to standing, then return to the start position. Repeat for reps, then switch sides.*

WIDE-GRIP ASSISTED PULL-UP
(Not Shown)

TARGETS: *Back, arms*
GET READY: *Set the assisted pull-up machine to 75% of your bodyweight. Grasp the bar with your palms facing forward and your hands as wide apart as possible.*
GO: *Pull your chin and chest toward the bar, pause, then control the descent.*

ROMANIAN DEADLIFT
(Not Shown)

TARGET: *Hamstrings*
GET READY: *Stand erect with your feet shoulder-width apart and your knees slightly bent. Grasp a dumbbell in each hand.*
GO: *Lean forward at the hips, sliding the weights down your legs until your hams and glutes tighten. Keep your back's natural arch as you return to the start.*

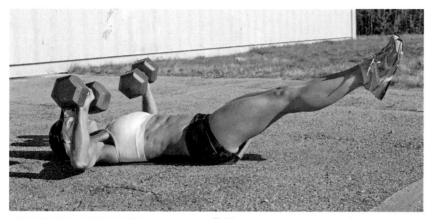

LYING LEG RAISE WITH DUMBBELLS

TARGETS: *Abs, chest*
GET READY: *Lie faceup on the floor and grasp a dumbbell in each hand, arms extended above your chest.*
GO: *Lift your feet off the floor, allowing only a slight bend in your knees, and raise your legs until they're nearly perpendicular to the floor. Slowly lower them and, without letting your heels touch down, perform a dumbbell press.*

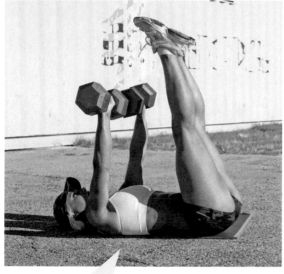

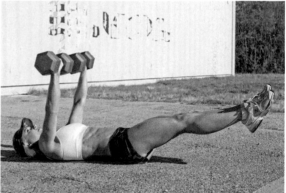

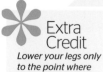

Extra Credit

Lower your legs only to the point where you can keep your low back pressed into the floor

ELEVATED PUSH-UP

TARGET: *Chest*
GET READY: *Place your toes up on a bench and your hands on the floor directly under your shoulders.*
GO: *Bend your elbows and lower your chest toward the floor. Keep your abs tight so your body forms a straight line from head to ankles. You can reverse the position by putting your feet on the floor and your hands on the bench, which reduces the pressure on your arms and shoulders.*

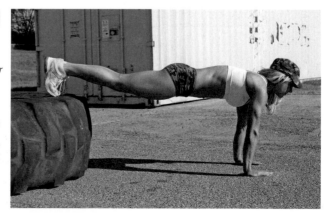

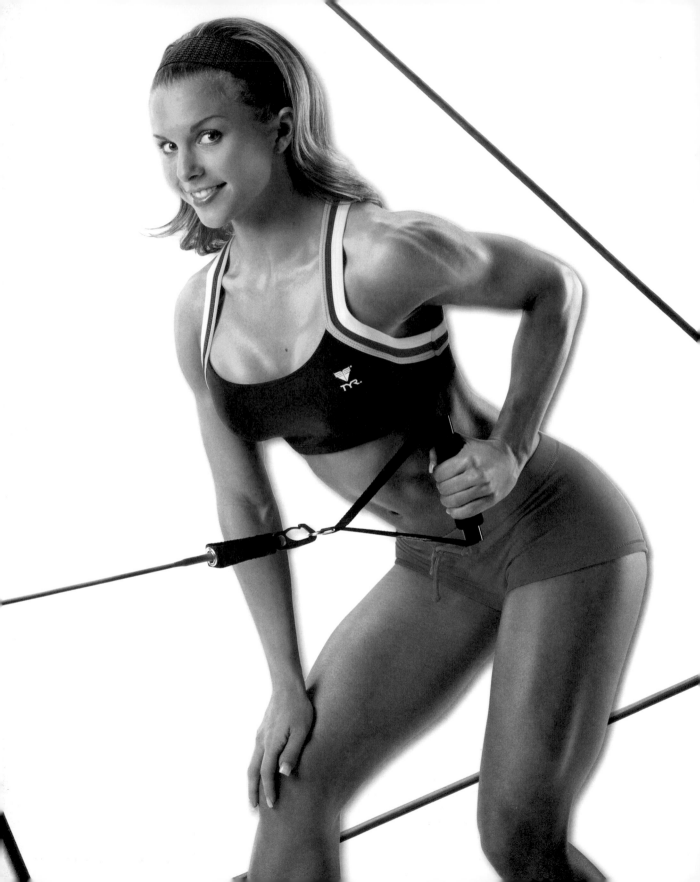

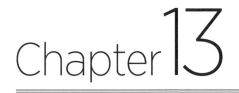
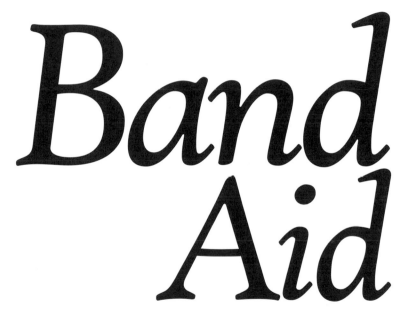

Band Aid

Whether you're a beginner or you've been training for years, exercise bands can make you stronger and more fit

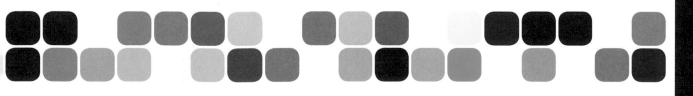

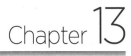

Chapter 13

We can just imagine the questions from our dedicated hardcore readers: Are exercise bands really effective? Aren't they the same oversized rubber bands used in '80s aerobics videos and physical therapy?

Yes, yes and yes. Bands have many uses and can be a valuable tool for anyone who's serious about gaining muscle definition and strength. If you're currently pursuing those worthy goals, you should incorporate them into your training regimen. We're not suggesting that you abandon weights, of course; we're merely recommending you add bands to your workouts.

If you're still skeptical, here's some science to back it up. In 2006, University of Wisconsin-La Crosse researchers reported in the *Journal of Strength & Conditioning Research* that trained subjects who added elastic bands to their routines experienced a significant increase in power. Similarly, subjects in a study conducted at Truman State University (Kirksville, Missouri) who trained with bands as well as free weights showed increased strength and power on the bench press compared to subjects who used only free weights.

Battle of the Bands

Here are four additional reasons bands are an effective tool and how they can help you in your quest for a better body:

1) **More resistance options** A 20-pound dumbbell weighs 20 pounds whether you hold it near your body or at arm's length. This isn't the case with exercise bands. Because of the physics of elastic, the tension increases as the band gets tauter, which means the resistance you'll feel at the start of a band press is markedly less than what you'll feel at the finish, when your arms are fully extended and the band is stretched nearly to its limit.

One benefit of this type of resistance is that as the difficulty increases, your body must call upon more fast-twitch muscle fibers, which are the strongest and most powerful. Athletes in almost every sport are incorporating bands into their training regimens to help them build power and strength.

Another advantage of resistance versatility is that it mimics the body's strength curve. Visualize a biceps curl, for example. From the point where your arm is fully extended to where your elbow forms about a 140-degree angle, your biceps is extremely weak. But as that angle narrows, your biceps becomes increasingly stronger. So when you use weights for biceps curls, you're limited to what you can lift during the first part of the curl. By the time you reach the point at which the biceps is stronger, the weight is too light to work the muscle to its maximum.

Since bands provide more resistance at the end of the curl, they work better to overload, and therefore strengthen, the muscle. In fact, people who use bands report feeling a "weird burn" in their muscles — which is the fast-twitch muscle fibers finally being used.

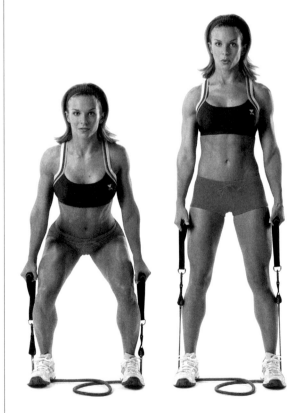

TARGET: *Legs*
GET READY: *Stand on the band with your feet near the ends. Grasp the handles just above your knees in a squat position.*
GO: *Pull the handles with you as you stand up in a slow and controlled manner, then return to the start. You can also attach bands to the ends of a barbell and squat with the bar.*

2) **Versatility in standard and functional training** Pop quiz: Why do you lie down when bench pressing? Because if you did the move standing up, it wouldn't be a chest exercise. The reason is that free weights work in only two directions: up and down. That's why you bend over when doing bent-over rows for back, stand up straight to do shoulder exercises and lie on your back to work your chest.

Bands don't rely on gravity to provide resistance, so you can use them not only in the vertical plane but also horizontally. It may be exhilarating to do a band bench press while standing, but the band is most useful in functional training. Have a fierce passion for your weekend softball league? Bands can strengthen your swing. Want to perfect your side kick to impress your sensei? Attach a band to your ankle and get kicking.

3) **No cheating** We see it all the time — people using a variety of motions to propel weights at the gym. They're not being fancy; they're cheating. Bands, on the other hand, are cheat-proof: No amount of pushing through your legs or swaying your back will change the fact that the band's resistance comes from its elasticity, not its weight. The only way to push a band is by involving more muscle fibers in the target area. The result? Better-defined muscles.

4) **Portability** You don't need a gym to work out with bands. While we generally recommend using them to augment your weight training, they're great if you're on vacation in a place without access to a weight room. You can plan an effective full-body training session right in your hotel room.

Band Together

Despite all the benefits of elastic resistance training, don't drop the weights altogether; we recommend that you use both. As you'll see in "Join the Band," adding band moves at the start and finish of your weight workouts can stretch your training and results to new heights.

Join the Band

⮑ There are two times in your weight routine when bands work great — at the beginning and end. Doing two sets of a band exercise as explosively as possible at the start of a workout offers two main benefits: 1) It serves as a great warm-up, and 2) it builds muscle power.

Doing two sets of a band exercise at the end of a workout specifically targets the muscle of interest and burns it out. For each major muscle group, try these two band exercises at the start and finish of each training session.

BODYPART	START EXERCISE[1]	FINISH EXERCISE[2]
Legs	Front Kick	Squat
Back	Standing Row	Straight-Arm Pulldown
Shoulders	Band Overhead Press	Band Lateral Raise
Chest	Punch Press	Band Flye
Triceps	Band Pushdown	One-Arm Overhead Extension
Biceps	Band Curl	Band Concentration Curl

[1] Do two sets of 5–8 reps: perform the positive portion of the rep as fast and explosively as possible.

[2] Perform two sets to failure, doing each rep in a slow and controlled manner.

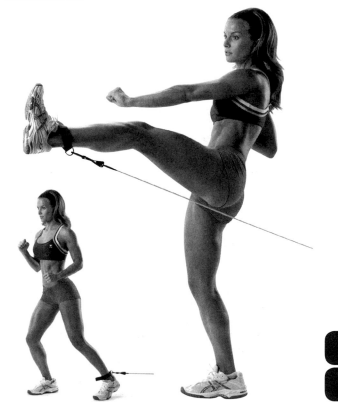

FRONT KICK

TARGET: *Legs*
GET READY: *Stand erect with your right foot forward in a fight stance. Affix one end of the band to your left ankle and the opposite end to a stable object behind you.*
GO: *Kick as high and explosively as possible with your left leg, and control the return. Repeat for reps, then switch sides.*

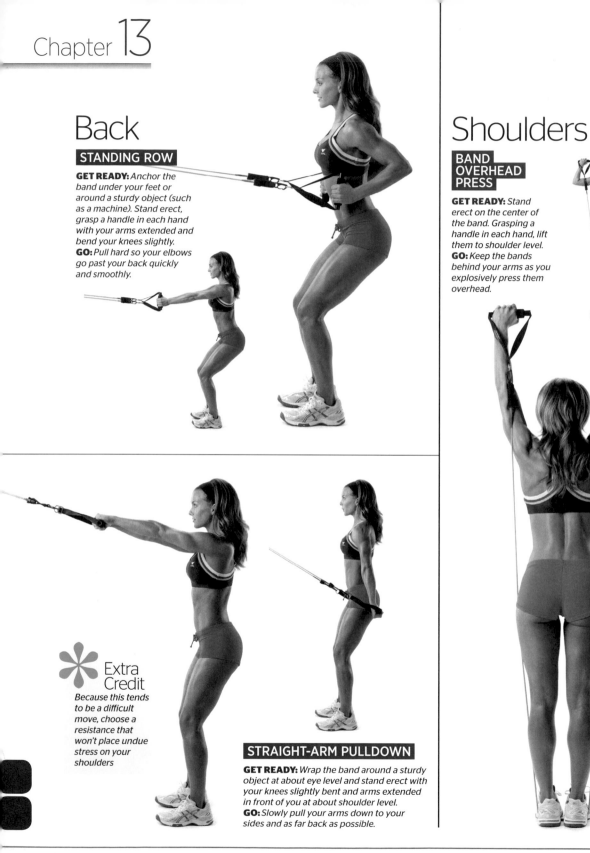

Chapter 13

Back

STANDING ROW

GET READY: *Anchor the band under your feet or around a sturdy object (such as a machine). Stand erect, grasp a handle in each hand with your arms extended and bend your knees slightly.*
GO: *Pull hard so your elbows go past your back quickly and smoothly.*

✳ Extra Credit

Because this tends to be a difficult move, choose a resistance that won't place undue stress on your shoulders

STRAIGHT-ARM PULLDOWN

GET READY: *Wrap the band around a sturdy object at about eye level and stand erect with your knees slightly bent and arms extended in front of you at about shoulder level.*
GO: *Slowly pull your arms down to your sides and as far back as possible.*

Shoulders

BAND OVERHEAD PRESS

GET READY: *Stand erect on the center of the band. Grasping a handle in each hand, lift them to shoulder level.*
GO: *Keep the bands behind your arms as you explosively press them overhead.*

Bonus Tip

You can add tension by widening your stance. Conversely, you can make the move easier by narrowing your base

BAND LATERAL RAISE

GET READY: *Stand erect on the center of the band with a handle in each hand near your thighs.*
GO: *Slowly lift your arms to just above parallel to the floor. Pause, then lower to just short of your arms touching your sides.*

Chest

BAND FLYE

GET READY: *Wrap the band around a sturdy object at chest level and turn sideways to it. Stand erect with the handle in your near hand and lift your arm straight out to your side.*
GO: *Pull your arm in front of you, crossing as far over your body as possible. Repeat for reps, then switch sides.*

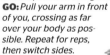

PUNCH PRESS

GET READY: *Wrap the band around a sturdy object at chest level and face away from it. Stand erect in a left-handed fight stance (right leg in front), knees bent slightly.*
GO: *Punch as explosively as possible with your left hand, keeping your arm at shoulder level. Repeat for reps, then switch sides.*

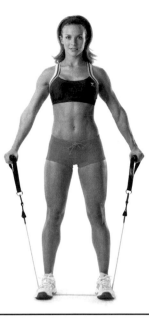

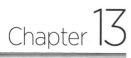

ONE-ARM OVERHEAD EXTENSION

GET READY: *Stand erect on the band with one foot near the end. Grasp the handle with your palm facing up, your upper arm alongside your ear and hand behind your head.*
GO: *Keeping your upper arm stationary, extend your arm overhead under control. Repeat for reps, then switch sides.*

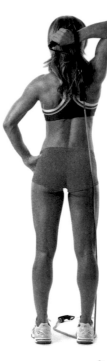

Triceps

BAND PUSHDOWN

GET READY: *Wrap the band around a tall, sturdy object and grasp a handle in each hand. Stand erect with your elbows bent 90 degrees and pinned to your sides, forearms parallel to the floor.*
GO: *Explosively press to full-arm extension, pause and control the return.*

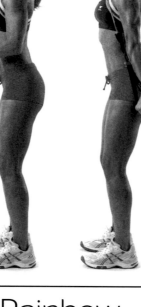

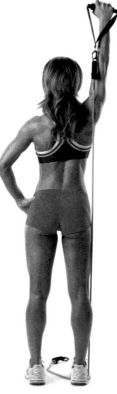

Rainbow Bands

➲ It's not just a marketing technique — the color of the band signifies its resistance. Here's a primer:

COLOR	RESISTANCE[1]	
Yellow	Extra light	
Green	Light	
Red	Medium	
Blue	Heavy	
Black	Extra heavy	

[1] In general, start with the least resistance. As a band becomes easier to manage, incrementally increase the resistance. If a jump from one color to the next is too much, use two bands of the same color.

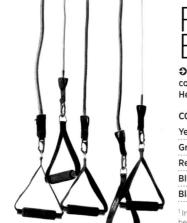

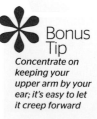

✳ Bonus Tip

Concentrate on keeping your upper arm by your ear; it's easy to let it creep forward

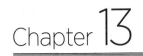

✳ Extra Credit

For variety, change your hand position so your palms face in or down to hit different areas of the biceps

Biceps

BAND CURL

GET READY: *Stand erect on the center of the band, feet shoulder-width apart. Grasp the handles in front of your thighs.*
GO: *Keeping your elbows pinned to your sides, curl the handles explosively toward your shoulders. Control the return.*

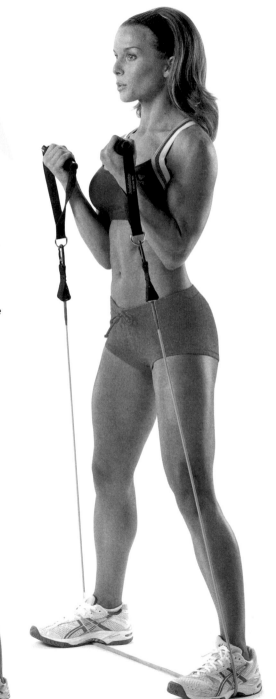

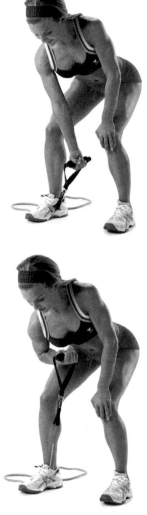

BAND CONCENTRATION CURL

GET READY: *Stand on the band with one foot near the end. Lean forward at the hips and grasp the handle nearest your foot.*
GO: *Slowly curl the handle toward your chest, keeping your elbow fixed near or inside your inner thigh, before lowering under control. Repeat for reps, then switch sides.*

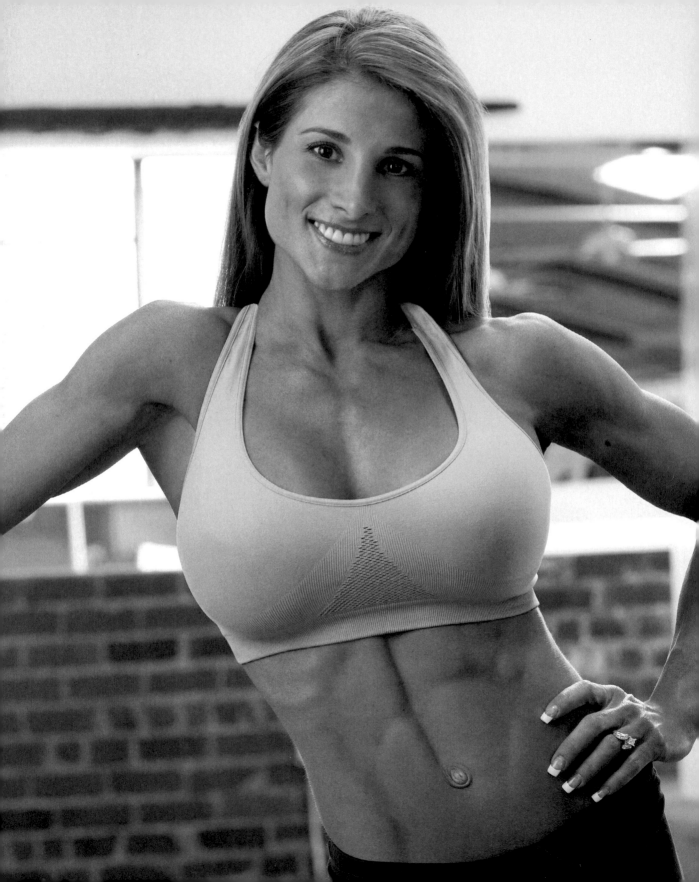

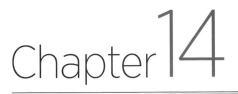

Chapter 14

The Arms You Want

No sleeves? No problem. Show off your arms anytime with our intense biceps and triceps workout

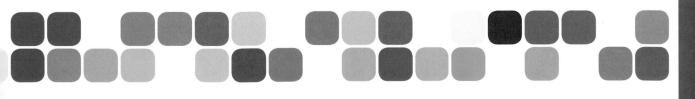

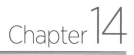
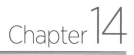

"Don't be afraid to lift heavy."
If IFBB figure pro Christine Pomponio-Pate can get you to remember one thing from this workout, it's that women shouldn't shy away from picking up bigger weights. "Women need to understand that the more muscle mass they have, the faster their metabolisms will be," she explains. "And we're built differently than men. So even if we go heavy, we won't get too big."

This last statement addresses the fear that many women have when they start a new biceps or triceps workout. Namely, they don't want "man arms." After 16 years of training, Christine is used to hearing this worry from gym enthusiasts.

"I understand this concern," she says. "And while I think women can be proud of having strong arms, there's a certain line [you don't want to cross] where it looks funny if you're too big, like if you're wearing an evening dress. I don't think I was ever to that point."

But this three-time Figure Olympia competitor wasn't afraid to push herself to the limits of her physique. "Honestly, if I could get really big naturally, I think I would've by now," she says. "But as women, we have physical limitations. I like being strong within those limits."

No Limits

Limitations, then, shouldn't be limiting. In fact, Christine subscribes heavily to the idea that women should listen to what their bodies tell them while exercising. As far as shaping your arms goes, if you're not getting results from your current routine, it's time to try something else.

"Learn what your body best reacts to," she says. "A lot of times I'll hear comments that I'm lifting heavier than most girls, but that's what works for me."

When it comes to what works for you, Christine suggests starting your arm routine with a weight that's light but not so light that you could fall asleep during the workout.

"Start off doing at least three sets with a weight you can lift for 8–10 reps," she says. "Once you get comfortable, you can switch things up. One week I'll go with heavy weights and fewer reps, and the next week I'll use lighter weights and do more reps."

Regardless of how you change up the variables in your workout, Christine insists that consistency is a key factor in gauging how successfully you'll achieve the goals you have for your arms, which begs the question: What kind of arms do you want?

"Some women have larger biceps and soft triceps," she says. "Others have the opposite. Find your weakness and work on it, striving for a total balance in your arms. Your biceps and triceps should be [equally strong, equally firm and] equally noticeable."

Having people notice your arms for just those reasons is what this whole workout is about.

The Routine

EXERCISE	SETS	REPS
One-Arm Reverse-Grip Pushdown	3–4	12–15 (each side)
Rope Hammer Curl	3	10–12
One-Arm High-Cable Curl	1	to failure (each side)
Standing Alternating Dumbbell Curl	3–4	8–10 (as heavy as you can)
Incline Lying Triceps Extension	2	12–15
Kickback	3–4	12

ONE-ARM HIGH-CABLE CURL

TARGET: *Biceps*
GET READY: *Stand erect alongside a high-pulley cable station, grasping a D-handle in your near hand. Take a step away to keep tension in the cable.*
GO: *Keeping your upper arm stationary just above parallel to the floor, curl the handle toward your ear, contracting your biceps at the top. Slowly return to the start position. Repeat for reps, then switch sides.*

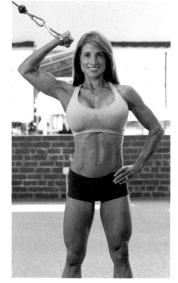

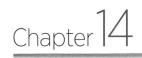
ONE-ARM REVERSE-GRIP PUSHDOWN

TARGET: *Triceps*

GET READY: *Stand erect in front of a high-pulley cable station and grasp the handle with an underhand grip. Take a step away from the weight stack.*

GO: *Keeping your upper arm by your side, straighten your elbow until your arm is fully extended. Slowly return to the start without allowing your forearm to go much past parallel to the floor at the top of the move. Repeat for reps, then switch sides.*

Bonus Tip

To move slightly heavier weight, use a palms-down grip

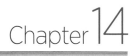
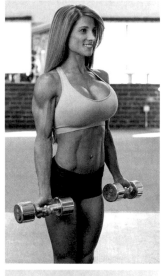

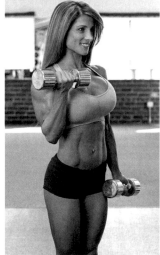

ROPE HAMMER CURL

TARGET: *Biceps*
GET READY: *Stand erect in front of a low-pulley cable station with a rope attached. Grasp both ends using a neutral grip and take a step back.*
GO: *Keeping your shoulders down and back, bend your elbows and curl the rope toward your chest, squeezing your biceps at the top. Keep your elbows at your sides; don't allow them to drift forward.*

✱ Extra Credit

For a stronger contraction at the top of the move, rotate your palms inward so they face your body

STANDING ALTERNATING DUMBBELL CURL

TARGET: *Biceps*
GET READY: *Stand erect with your feet hip-width apart, holding dumbbells in front of your thighs with your palms facing forward.*
GO: *Keeping your stronger arm down at your side, curl with your weaker arm first, making sure your elbow stays pinned alongside your ribcage. Lower the weight, then curl with your other arm. Keep your shoulders down and back; only your forearms move throughout the exercise.*

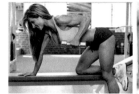

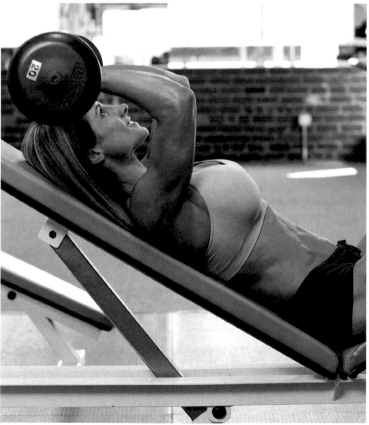

KICKBACK

TARGET: *Triceps*

GET READY: *Place one hand and the same-side knee on a flat bench. Keep your shoulders, back and hips flat and parallel to the floor. Grasp a dumbbell in your free hand and raise your upper arm alongside your torso.*

GO: *Keeping your upper arm stationary, extend your elbow until your arm is straight and parallel to the floor. Slowly return to the start. Repeat for reps, then switch sides.*

✳ Bonus Tip

Don't swing the weight up or hunch your back to extend your arm. Use a slow, controlled movement

INCLINE LYING TRICEPS EXTENSION

TARGET: *Triceps*

GET READY: *Lie faceup on an incline bench set to 45 degrees and grasp a fixed-weight bar or barbell with an overhand, shoulder-width grip.*

GO: *Press the bar toward the ceiling over your collarbones. Keeping your upper arms in place, bend your elbows to lower the bar to just above your forehead without letting your elbows flare out. Extend your arms to press the bar back toward the ceiling.*

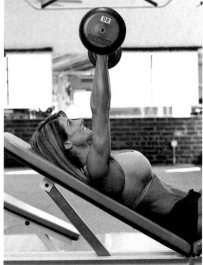

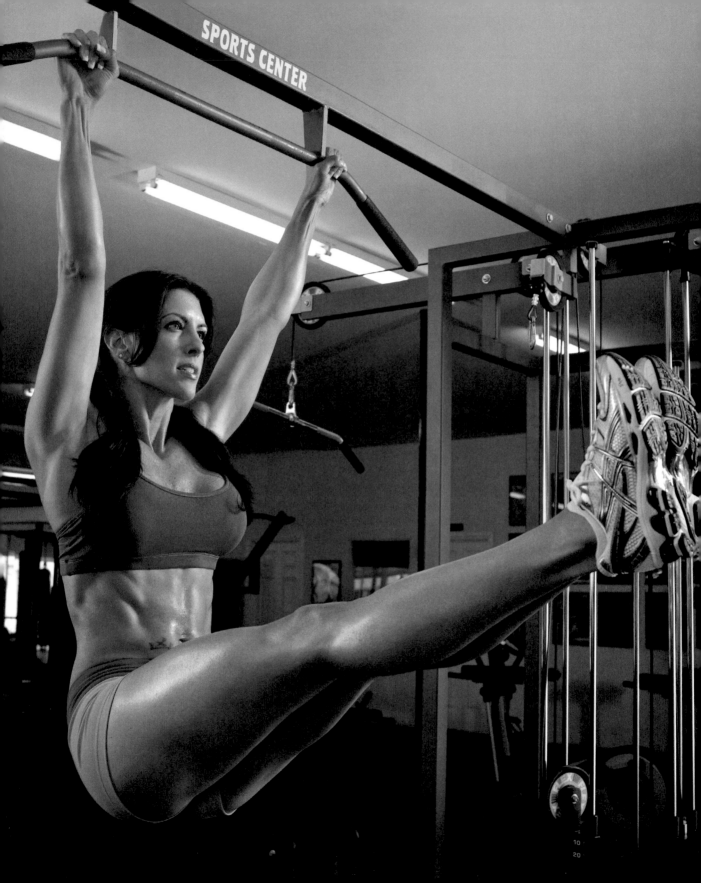

Build Your Own Abs

Like anything else, sculpting an amazing midsection takes commitment, dedication and knowledge. We can help with that last part

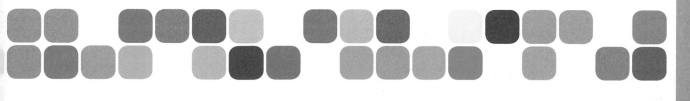

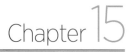
Quick — pick a bodypart you want to improve. Okay, now pick another one. Abs, right? First and foremost, showcasing a toned midsection takes the right diet and the right type of cardio. But it also means knowing the ins and outs of ab training, from the exercises to the frequency to how fast or slow to perform the repetitions. Here, we break down everything you need to know about training abs to help you sculpt the core you've always wanted.

The Workout

Putting together an ab program is very simple, as long as you remember one thing: There's a strict order to the exercises: Always choose lower-ab moves first, then upper, then obliques and finally core. This is the Weider Principle of priority training, where you focus on weaker areas by doing the hardest exercises first. You can substitute any exercise that works the same region when you design your own workout. Here are three sample routines to get you started.

GROUP 1
LOWER ABS

Sample Ab Day: Bodyweight

AB REGION	EXERCISE	SETS/REPS
Lower Abs	Hip Thrust	2–3/failure
Upper Abs	Decline Crunch	2–3/10–15
Obliques	Reaching Crossover Crunch	2–3/15–20
Core	Plank	2–3/failure

Sample Ab Day: Weighted

AB REGION	EXERCISE	SETS/REPS
Lower Abs	Weighted Hanging Knee Raise	2–3/failure
Upper Abs	Weighted Crunch	2–3/10–15
Obliques	Standing Oblique Cable Crunch	2–3/15–20
Core	Dumbbell Woodchopper	2–3/15–20

Sample Ab Day: Exercise Ball

AB REGION	EXERCISE	SETS/REPS
Lower Abs	Exercise-Ball Roll-In	2–3/failure
Upper Abs	Exercise-Ball Crunch	2–3/10–15
Obliques	Exercise-Ball Roll-In to the Side	2–3/15–20
Core	Exercise-Ball Pass	2–3/15–20

RECOMMENDED EXERCISES:
EXERCISE-BALL REVERSE CRUNCH
HANGING KNEE RAISE
HANGING LEG RAISE
HIP THRUST
REVERSE CRUNCH
EXERCISE-BALL ROLL-IN

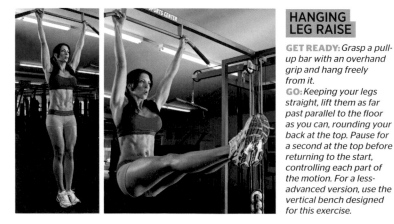

HANGING LEG RAISE

GET READY: *Grasp a pull-up bar with an overhand grip and hang freely from it.*
GO: *Keeping your legs straight, lift them as far past parallel to the floor as you can, rounding your back at the top. Pause for a second at the top before returning to the start, controlling each part of the motion. For a less-advanced version, use the vertical bench designed for this exercise.*

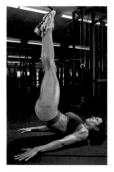

HIP THRUST

GET READY: *Lie faceup on the floor. Bend your hips to a 90-degree angle so your legs point toward the ceiling. Place your hands at your sides for support.*
GO: *Keeping your shoulders and head on the floor, squeeze your abs to lift your hips and glutes off the floor. Hold the peak-contracted position for a moment before returning to the start.*

GROUP 2
UPPER ABS

RECOMMENDED EXERCISES: CABLE CRUNCH DECLINE CRUNCH DUMBBELL V-SIT EXERCISE-BALL CRUNCH STRAIGHT-LEG CRUNCH V-UP WEIGHTED CRUNCH

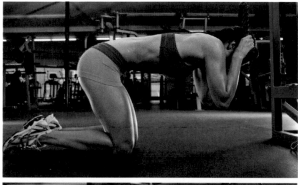

CABLE CRUNCH

GET READY: *Attach a rope to a high-pulley cable and kneel facing the weight stack. Grasp the rope with both hands, bend your elbows and pull your hands down to about ear level.* **GO:** *Bend at the hips and, keeping your lower back parallel to the floor and hands locked alongside your head, curl your elbows toward your knees. Squeeze your abs and return to the start.*

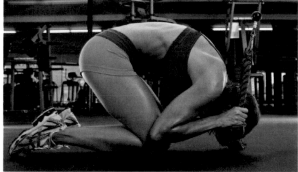

✳ Bonus Tip
Keep the rest periods between sets short — one minute or less. Abs are considered postural muscles, used primarily to keep you standing upright, so they recover more quickly than other muscle groups

WEIGHTED CRUNCH

GET READY: *Lie faceup on the floor, bend your knees and place your feet flat on the floor. Hold a weight plate at your chest with both hands.* **GO:** *Keeping your eyes focused on the ceiling, lift your shoulders off the floor. Squeeze your abs and return to the start, keeping your neck in a neutral position.*

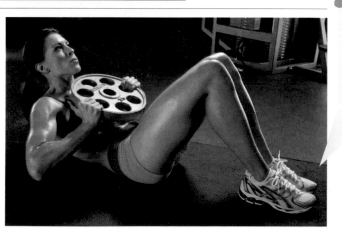

✳ Extra Credit
Using weights won't thicken your waist because abs have the capacity to grow only so big. Instead, you're likely to carve out the definition you're looking for

GROUP 3
OBLIQUES

RECOMMENDED EXERCISES:

CROSSOVER CRUNCH
OBLIQUE CRUNCH
REACHING CROSSOVER CRUNCH
RUSSIAN TWIST

STANDING DUMBBELL OBLIQUE CRUNCH
STANDING OBLIQUE CABLE CRUNCH
EXERCISE-BALL ROLL-IN TO THE SIDE

RUSSIAN TWIST

GET READY: *Sit on a decline sit-up bench and lean back so your abs are engaged. Grasp a dumbbell with both hands using a neutral grip and extend your arms in front of you.* **GO:** *Keeping your elbows locked and back flat, rotate your torso to the left until your arms are parallel to the floor. Pause, then return to the start. Repeat the movement to the right; that's one rep.*

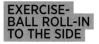

Bonus Tip
Just like any other muscle, abs must be broken down before they grow. To tax the muscle, you must provide sufficient overload. For certain exercises, you may be able to do too many reps to be effective. That's when you need to add weight

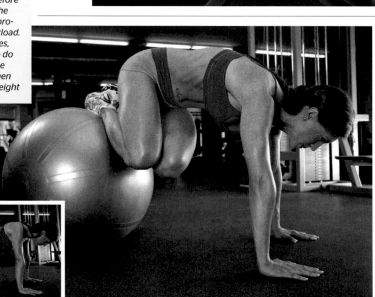

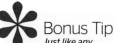

EXERCISE-BALL ROLL-IN TO THE SIDE

GET READY: *Start in push-up position, hands shoulder-width apart on the floor and your shins atop an exercise ball.* **GO:** *Keep your legs together as you bend your knees and draw them toward your right elbow, rolling the ball forward as you do so. Pause, then extend your legs to return to the start. Roll the ball toward your left elbow to complete one rep.*

GROUP 4
CORE

RECOMMENDED EXERCISES: CABLE WOODCHOPPER   EXERCISE-BALL PASS   PLANK
DUMBBELL WOODCHOPPER   EXERCISE-BALL ROLL-OUT   SCISSOR KICK
LYING LEG RAISE

PLANK

GET READY: *Get into push-up position but with your elbows bent 90 degrees, forearms on the floor about shoulder-width apart.*
GO: *Tighten your core, pulling your belly button toward your spine, and keep your back flat. Allow only your forearms and toes to support your bodyweight. Hold the position to failure.*

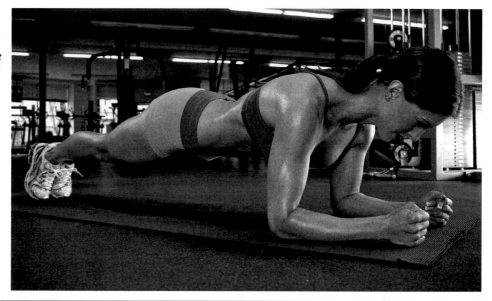

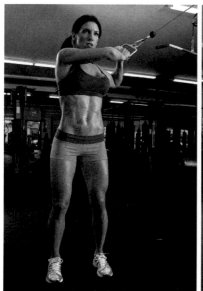
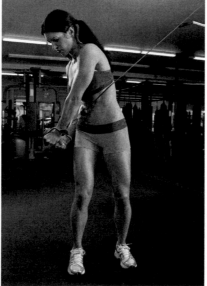

CABLE WOODCHOPPER

GET READY: *Attach a D-handle to a high-pulley cable. Stand alongside and an arm's length away from the weight stack. Grasp the handle with both hands above your left shoulder as if you're holding a baseball bat.*
GO: *Pull the handle across your body to your right hip, pause and return under control. Repeat for reps, then switch sides.*

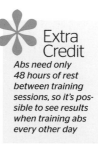

Extra Credit

Abs need only 48 hours of rest between training sessions, so it's possible to see results when training abs every other day

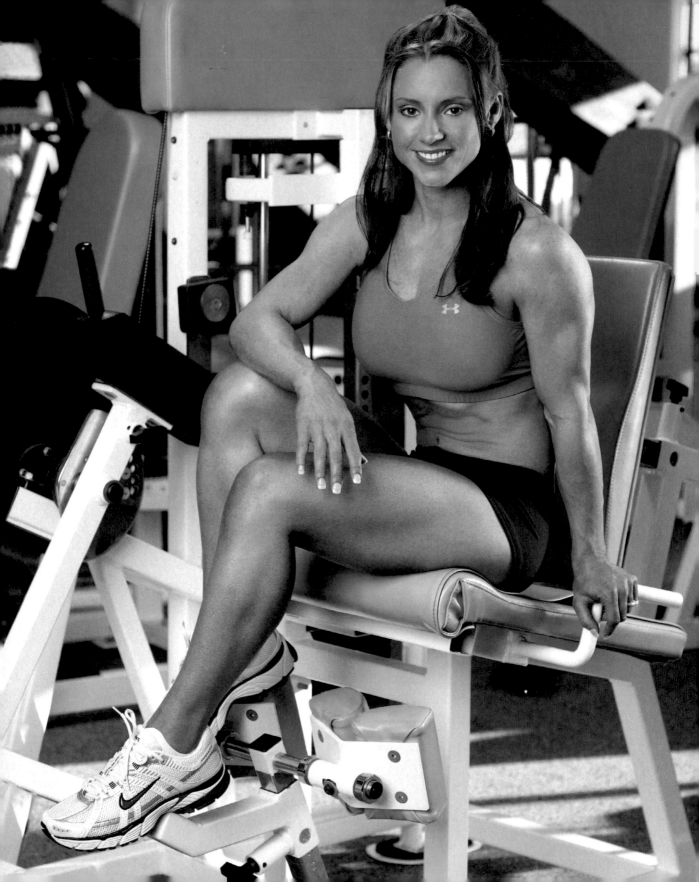

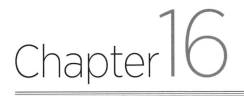

Chapter 16

Perfect Harmony

This targeted leg routine may be just what your thighs and glutes have been waiting for

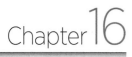
Figure competitors are the micromanagers of the fitness set. Their goal is to shape each bodypart so the end result, the gestalt of the final product, is a perfect harmony of well-conditioned parts. To those nonprofessionals aspiring to a similar balance, it may seem as if these women are blessed with agreeable bodies whose arms, backs, legs and shoulders all reach their peaks at the same time.

Jennifer Gates, who won the 2008 Figure Olympia, has some good news for you: When it comes to training legs, she works extra-hard to ensure they make the grade. She knows this is a stubborn area for most women, and that losing fat and adding muscle there is especially difficult. "My legs are usually the last bodypart to come in before a show," she admits.

The key to getting your legs to "come in" is to know what you want from them in the first place. Her hamstrings aside, Jennifer — a pediatric nurse and mother of two — believes she has all the muscle size she needs in her legs, so she focuses most of her effort on adding shape and definition to what she has already built. "I don't go heavy with any of my leg exercises, except hamstrings," she says. In fact, awhile back she added a second leg day to her schedule in an effort to tighten up her hams. "I do six sets of stiff-legged deadlifts," she explains.

For those who feel their legs have enough muscle, Jennifer recommends a high-rep, lightweight workout in which you maintain a high level of intensity. "I keep my pace with leg training fast because it keeps my heart rate up and I get a really good burn this way."

She likes to start off her leg workout with two warm-up sets of leg extensions before moving on to her working sets. Even though she prefers to keep the pace quick, she's careful not to compromise form or control, which can minimize the actual work her legs get from the exercise.

This is especially important with a move such as the incline dumbbell lying leg curl. The balance required to do this exercise makes it particularly cumbersome for first-timers, but once mastered, it's a great move for strengthening the core as well as the hamstrings. Jennifer believes she gets a better workout from this variation than from the leg curl machine.

The plié squat is another regular move in her leg routine that has paid off for her. The exercise hits the quads, hamstrings and glutes, and has been instrumental in helping her shape and tone these areas.

Then there's her cardio routine, an equally vital component in the development of her legs. When preparing for a show, Jennifer does cardio twice a day for about 45 minutes. "I run bleachers, do sprints and walk the treadmill on an incline," she says.

Yet even with this intensive regimen, which she usually starts 12 weeks before a competition, changes must be made often if her legs are being stubborn. To begin with, Jennifer always trains with a partner, someone who can push her and help her through any rough spots. If that's not enough, she'll switch her workouts around. "I'll either do more cardio or something different altogether," she says. "Instead of walking on the treadmill, I'll switch to the StepMill."

By listening to her body and observing the results of her time in the gym, Jennifer is better able to create the perfect harmony of parts that the figure stage demands. It's a lesson with a lot to teach anyone who spends serious time building a better body.

The Routine

EXERCISE	SETS	REPS
Plié Squat	4	20
Incline Dumbbell Lying Leg Curl	4	12–15
Bench Step-Up	4	50
Leg Extension	4	20

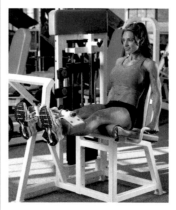

LEG EXTENSION

TARGET: *Quads*
GET READY: *Sit squarely in the machine with your knees in line with the axis of rotation and your feet under the ankle pads.*
GO: *With your toes pointed straight, extend your legs as high as you can while keeping your back and hips flush against the seat. Squeeze your quads hard at the top, then slowly lower the weight until just short of the stack touching down.*

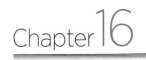

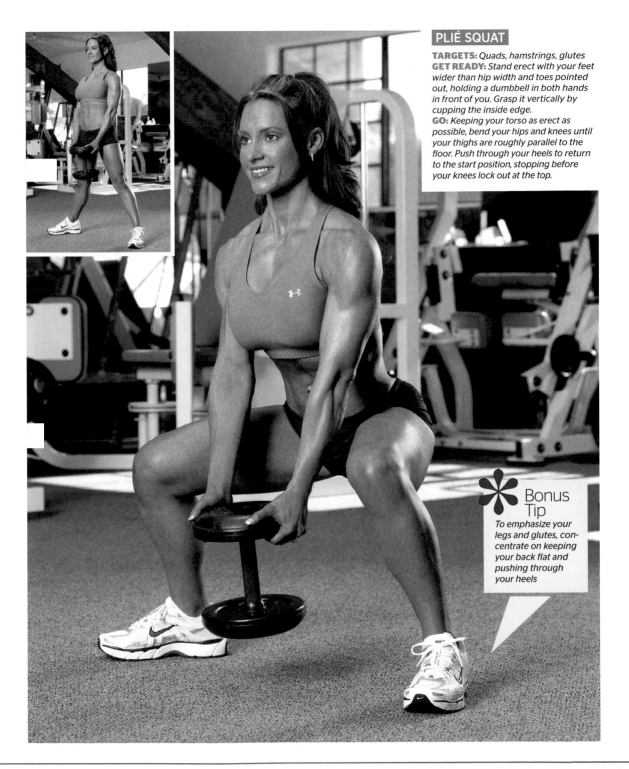

PLIÉ SQUAT

TARGETS: *Quads, hamstrings, glutes*
GET READY: *Stand erect with your feet wider than hip width and toes pointed out, holding a dumbbell in both hands in front of you. Grasp it vertically by cupping the inside edge.*
GO: *Keeping your torso as erect as possible, bend your hips and knees until your thighs are roughly parallel to the floor. Push through your heels to return to the start position, stopping before your knees lock out at the top.*

Bonus Tip
To emphasize your legs and glutes, concentrate on keeping your back flat and pushing through your heels

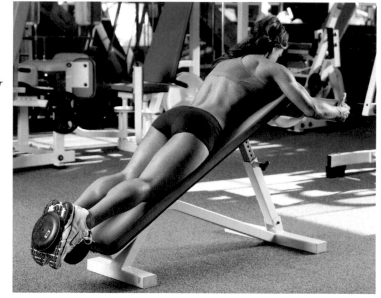

INCLINE DUMBBELL LYING LEG CURL

TARGETS: *Hamstrings, glutes*

GET READY: *Lie facedown on a decline bench with your head at the top and your knees slightly bent. Have a spotter place a dumbbell between your feet, then squeeze them together to hold the weight in place.*

GO: *Keeping your body flat on the bench, curl your feet as high as possible by contracting your hamstrings. Hold for a brief count, then slowly lower the weight.*

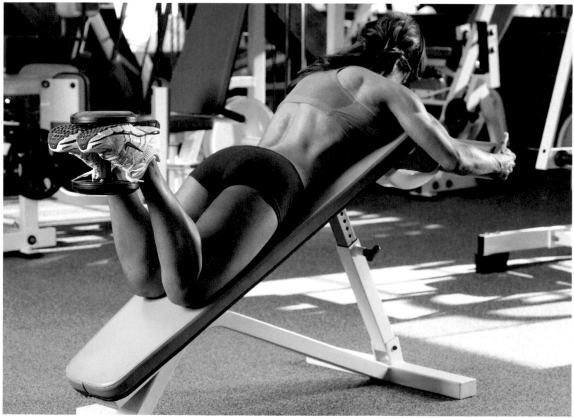

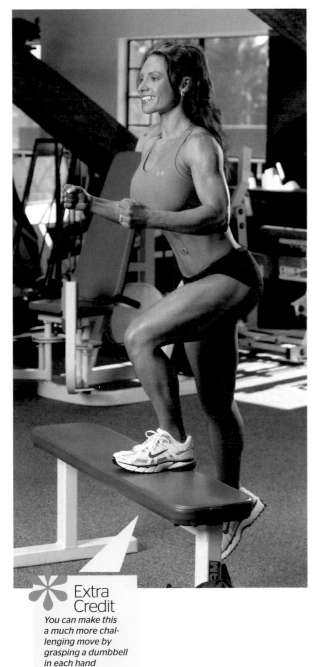

Extra Credit

You can make this a much more challenging move by grasping a dumbbell in each hand

BENCH STEP-UP

TARGETS: *Quads, hamstrings, glutes*

GET READY: *Stand erect in front of a bench, block or step and place one foot on it. The movement is shown without weight, but you can also grasp a dumbbell in each hand for added resistance.*

GO: *Press through your front heel to raise your body and bring your back foot onto the bench. Bend your front knee to return just your back foot to the floor. Repeat for reps, then switch sides.*

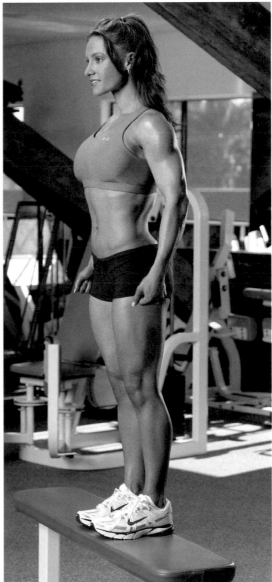

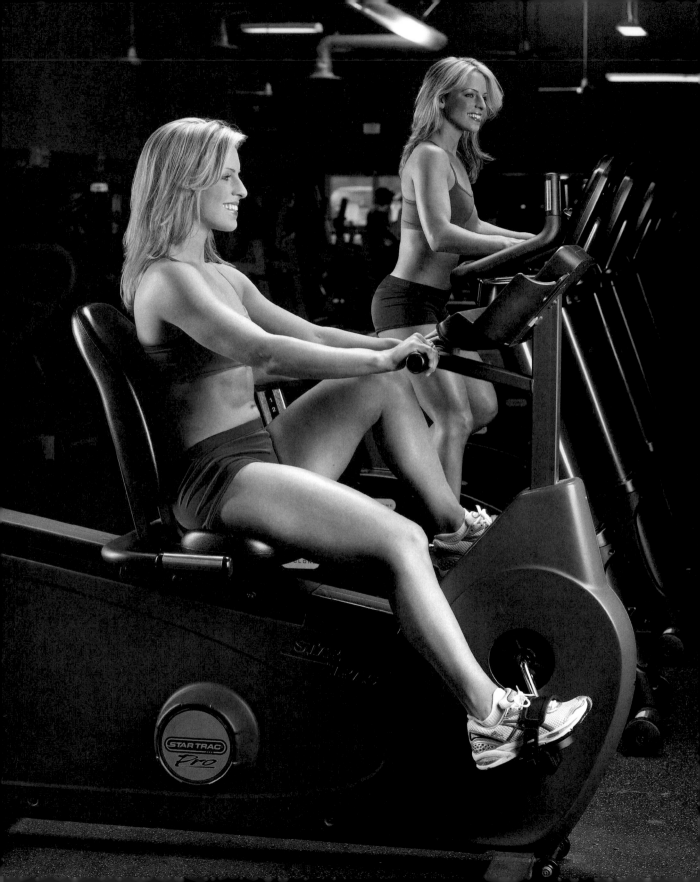

Chapter 17

Cardio Match-Up

Who says you have to spend forever on the treadmill to get lean? By piecing together a few high-intensity intervals, you can crank your fat-fighting machinery into overdrive

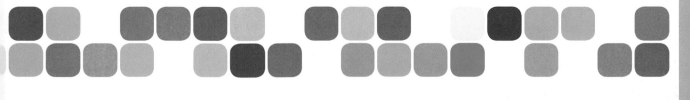

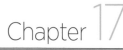
Ninety minutes of cardio:

Before you flip the page in fear and/or disgust, allow us to clarify. We're not pinning your fat-fighting efforts to a single, monotonous session of treadmill torture. Cruel and unusual isn't our strong suit, and we wouldn't expect you to do something we weren't prepared to do ourselves. Instead, we're providing you with nine distinct 10-minute cardio sessions that you can mix and match at your discretion to melt away unwanted bodyfat.

But we should warn you: These aren't the types of routines you can just stride through at a leisurely pace to the musical stylings of Bob Marley. These are leave-it-all-in-the-gym, fat-blasting bouts of exercise that will have you sucking wind.

Why the breakneck pace? For one thing, we're running out of space in our offices with the influx of research on how high-intensity interval training (HIIT) is leaving traditional steady-state cardio in its dust. HIIT, though performed in shorter, segmented bursts, burns more calories because of the greater exertion, and — this is the real bonus — it keeps your body in fat-burning mode long after you've undone the laces on your running shoes. That metabolic benefit, known as excess post-exercise oxygen consumption (EPOC), is the chief payout of this type of training.

Here, we offer nine different HIIT workouts, each lasting 10 minutes. While we usually prescribe 20–40 minutes worth of cardio to keep eating into your fat stores, these programs can be intermingled in any order and for any length of time that you see fit. For example, instead of 30 minutes of interval work on the bike, you can hit the rower, treadmill and StepMill for 10 minutes apiece. Thirty minutes is 30 minutes, and your body will respond accordingly.

This is especially good for those of you who have short attention spans because this departure from the yawn-inducing practices of cardio past will keep you focused from start to finish. Just make sure you warm up, cool down and stretch before admiring the fruits of your labor in the mirror.

String Training

Weave together as many of the following nine workouts as you'd like to create a varied, high-intensity cardio program. Shifting between these routines helps you burn more total calories in a shorter period than traditional steady-state training and stokes your metabolic fire to continue burning fat long after you leave the gym. Of course, if you find that a particular workout is more enjoyable or effective, feel free to keep at it by adding as many intervals as you'd like. As your body adapts, step up the intensity by raising the resistance or incline, or by making your high-intensity bouts longer and recovery bouts shorter.

For all of these programs, you'll work on a scale of perceived exertion, or PE. On a scale of 1–10, with 10 being high, the PE scale is a guide to gauge your effort level. Obviously, the scale isn't exact; there are numerous factors to consider when it comes to how hard someone is working, but use it as a basic means to determine your work level.

Be sure to warm up for at least five minutes before starting any of these programs, and set aside at least 5–10 minutes afterward to stretch.

Bonus Tip

Keep yourself moving in the gym by combining three (or more) pieces of cardio equipment

Mix & Match
SAMPLE WORKOUT

EQUIPMENT	PROGRAM
Treadmill	No. 1
Recumbent Bike	No. 2
Elliptical Trainer	No. 3

These three programs — outlined on the next page — offer just one of many cardio combos you can use to burn bodyfat.

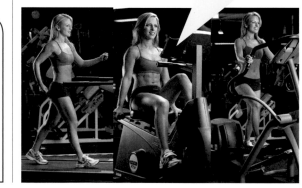

1) Treadmill

This is no ordinary conveyor-belt joyride. Begin with a one-minute walk before moving into a quicker stride. From there, you hit a minute-long sprint before repeating the cycle twice more.

TIME/PACE	PE (INTENSITY)
1 min. walk	2
1 min. stride	6
1 min. sprint	9
1 min. walk	2
1 min. stride	6
1 min. sprint	9
1 min. walk	2
1 min. stride	6
2 min. sprint	10

2) Recumbent Bike

The seated bicycle is a great leg-shaper and calorie-burner. This routine varies between high and low intensity — no middle ground to plod through here. For your sprints, adjust the resistance so it's a difficult minute, since cranking away with little to no resistance is only going to make you look silly, anyway.

TIME/PACE	PE (INTENSITY)
1 min. slow ride	3
1 min. sprint	10
1 min. slow ride	3
1 min. sprint	10
1 min. slow ride	3
1 min. sprint	10
1 min. slow ride	3
1 min. sprint	10
1 min. slow ride	3
1 min. sprint	10

3) Elliptical Trainer

The elliptical machine is a great cardio tool because you can adjust the incline and resistance fairly easily. This program provides guidelines that are more resistance-specific, but adjusting to a higher incline as you progress will allow you to continue making gains with this piece of equipment.

TIME/RESISTANCE	PE (INTENSITY)
2 min. medium resistance	5
30 sec. low resistance	2
1 min. high resistance	10
30 sec. low resistance	2
2 min. medium resistance	5
30 sec. low resistance	2
1 min. high resistance	10
30 sec. low resistance	2
2 min. medium resistance	5

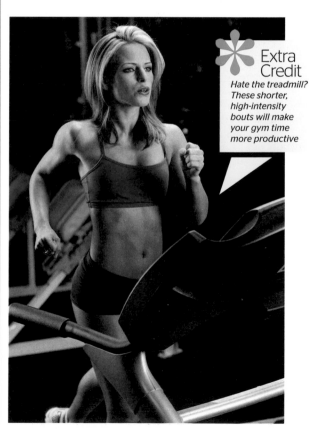

Extra Credit

Hate the treadmill? These shorter, high-intensity bouts will make your gym time more productive

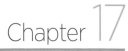

4) Incline Treadmill

This is a treadmill routine like Workout No. 1, but this time you'll set the incline to 5% to further engage your calves, glutes and hamstrings. Each interval features a short, uphill sprint followed by complete rest. For your rest periods, step onto the side rails adjacent to the belt or carefully step off the treadmill.

TIME/PACE	PE (INTENSITY)
15 sec. uphill sprint	10
15 sec. rest	—
30 sec. uphill sprint	10
30 sec. rest	—
45 sec. uphill sprint	10
45 sec. rest	—
1 min. uphill sprint	10
1 min. rest	—
1 min. uphill sprint	10
1 min. rest	—
1 min. uphill sprint	10
1 min. rest	—
1 min. uphill sprint	10

5) Rower

This underused piece of gym equipment provides total-body training and thus great fat-burning benefits. While many are digital, you can increase or decrease the resistance on most machines by adjusting the dial on the wheel itself. Be sure to use your legs to initiate each pull.

TIME/PACE	PE (INTENSITY)
5 min. slow row	3
1 min. fast row	8
1 min. slow row	4
1 min. fast row	9
1 min. slow row	5
1 min. fast row	10

6) Treadmill

At first glance, this treadmill routine may seem relatively easy. However, the longer jogs definitely put your fitness to the test. Again, the more accurately you can gauge your perceived level of exertion, the more productive your workout will be.

TIME/PACE	PE (INTENSITY)
2 min. easy jog	5
2 min. walk	1
2 min. easy jog	5
2 min. walk	1
2 min. easy jog	5

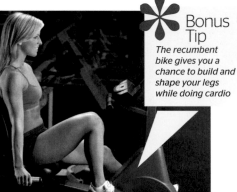

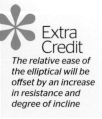

Bonus Tip

The recumbent bike gives you a chance to build and shape your legs while doing cardio

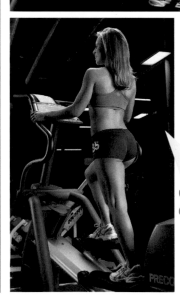

Extra Credit

The relative ease of the elliptical will be offset by an increase in resistance and degree of incline

7) Rower

This time on the rower, blast your body with three-minute "sprints" paced alternately by a single minute of slow rowing. Again, don't allow your arms to dominate the cadence — use your legs to create a steady, balanced pace.

TIME/PACE	PE (INTENSITY)
1 min. slow row	4
3 min. fast row	7
1 min. slow row	4
3 min. fast row	7
2 min. slow row	5

8) Bike

You'll use three speeds during this routine: slow, fast and sprint. Your fast ride should be from the seat; however, by "out of saddle" we mean up off the seat à la Lance Armstrong heading for the finish line.

TIME/PACE	PE (INTENSITY)
30 sec. slow ride	3
30 sec. fast ride	8
30 sec. out of saddle	10
30 sec. slow ride	3
30 sec. fast ride	8
30 sec. out of saddle	10
30 sec. slow ride	3
30 sec. fast ride	8
30 sec. out of saddle	10
30 sec. slow ride	3
30 sec. fast ride	8
30 sec. out of saddle	10
30 sec. slow ride	3
30 sec. fast ride	8
30 sec. out of saddle	10
30 sec. slow ride	3
30 sec. fast ride	8
30 sec. out of saddle	10
1 min. slow ride	3

9) StepMill

Many professional fitness and figure athletes are fans of the StepMill because it burns fat and enhances the look of their legs.

TIME/PACE	PE (INTENSITY)
15 sec. slow climb	2
30 sec. fast climb	7
15 sec. slow climb	2
30 sec. fast climb	7
15 sec. slow climb	2
30 sec. fast climb	7
15 sec. slow climb	2
30 sec. fast climb	7
1 min. slow climb	3
1 min. fast climb	8
15 sec. slow climb	2
30 sec. fast climb	7
15 sec. slow climb	2
30 sec. fast climb	7
15 sec. slow climb	2
30 sec. fast climb	7
15 sec. slow climb	2
30 sec. fast climb	7
1 min. slow climb	3
1 min. fast climb	8

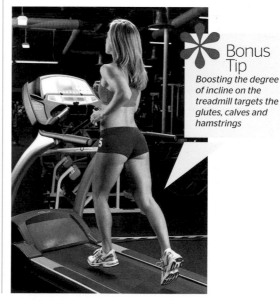

Bonus Tip

Boosting the degree of incline on the treadmill targets the glutes, calves and hamstrings

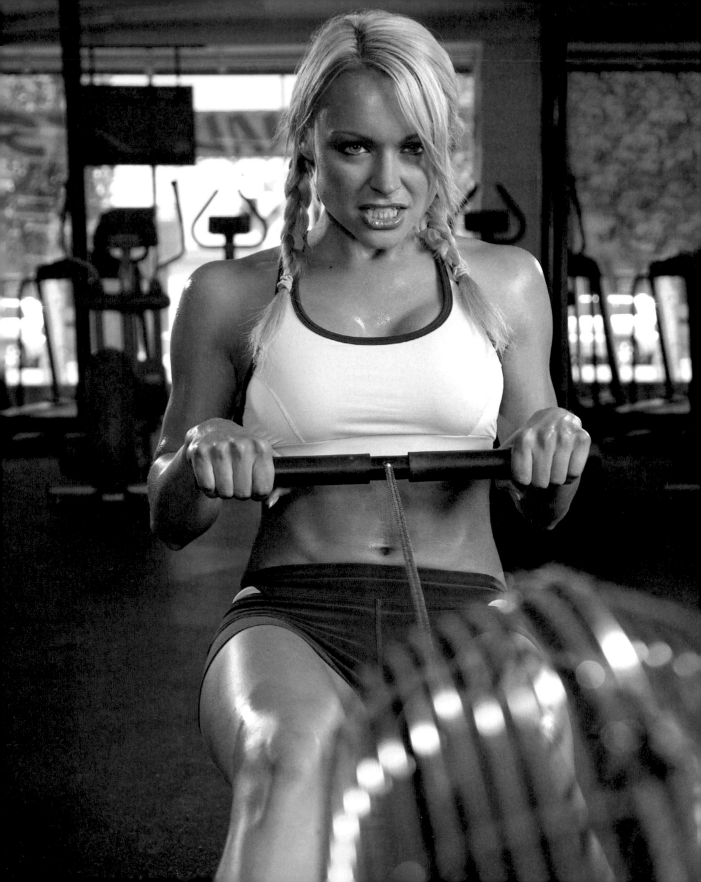

Super Intervals

Short and brutal sprints can cut fat, build muscle and radically reduce your workout time — if you can handle them

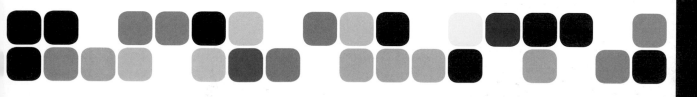

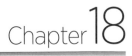
Ginger Bryant was never petite. At 6'1" and 165 pounds, she starred on the 1998 NAIA champion volleyball team at Union University (Jackson, Tennessee). Ten years out of college, she looked in the mirror and saw 260 pounds staring back. "I gained nearly 100 pounds — I was really big," said the fitness-club manager. "So in March 2008 I cleaned up my diet, lifted weights and hit the treadmill, but I lost only 15 pounds in seven months. It was frustrating."

That started to change in October, and by May Bryant had gone from a size 20 to a size 10. She lost 70 pounds, down to 181, and was aiming for 165 by July. "It was magic," she says. "The weight just fell off. I was leaning out overnight and everyone noticed. People would ask, 'What are you doing?' And I'd tell them I was working out less — from an hour on the treadmill down to 20 minutes on the bike." Her secret? Bryant ditched the long, slow cardio sessions for a program of 30-second all-out sprints.

And she's not the only one. San Francisco personal trainer Sarah Harding Traverso claims that going shorter and harder helped her win the 2006 Ms. Fitness USA crown, stay strong during her five years as a Cirque du Soleil acrobat and reduce her exercise-induced asthma. Nicole Avellina, 2005 Ms. Fitness USA champion and a former arena football cheerleader from Central Islip, New York, lost 30 pounds of stubborn post-pregnancy weight in five months by doing sprint work for just an hour a week. "It's 30 seconds of terror," she says. "But it's over quickly and I have more energy. I even sleep better at night."

This is no run-of-the-mill interval; it's an all-out, 30-second, fight-or-flight experience that boosts your heart rate through the roof. Do eight of these super-intervals, recovering for 60–120 seconds between each, and you'll enjoy cardio and strength gains, and rapid fat loss — all with just four minutes of sprints within 20 minutes of total workout time. And the system works for everyone, from bodybuilders to marathon runners.

Backed by Research

Superintervals build fitness through a phenomenon called the stress adaptation response, in which the human body adapts to stress by getting stronger. In the case of superintervals, the body is pushed beyond its aerobic threshold, so it upgrades its oxygen-processing system with new capillaries and develops a higher tolerance to the buildup of lactic acid.

"The effect works for everyone of every age," says Leonard A. Kaminsky, PhD, director of the clinical exercise physiology program at the Ball State University (Muncie, Indiana) human performance lab and editor of the exercise guidelines manual of the American College of Sports Medicine. Plenty of studies have proven how effective intervals can be. In a 2006 *Journal of Physiology* study from McMaster

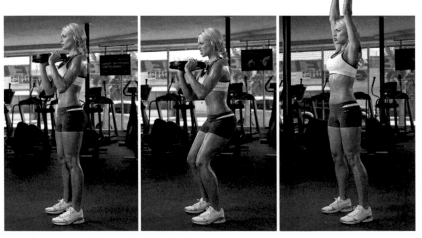

PUSH-PRESS

TARGETS: *Legs, shoulders*
GET READY: *Stand erect with your feet wider than shoulder width, holding a weight plate at your collarbones with both hands.*
GO: *Bend your hips and knees to descend into a half-squat. Explode up through your legs and push the weight overhead, then return to the start. Think of this as three separate moves: dip, drive and return.*

University (Hamilton, Ontario, Canada), researchers found that trained subjects who performed 20 minutes of cycling intervals per day developed the same fitness levels as those who rode at a moderate pace for two hours a day — six times as long!

Serious athletes benefit, too. In a 2005 study from Waikato Institute of Technology (Hamilton, New Zealand), scientists found that intervals boosted the performance of bike racers in midseason form. After 8–12 sessions, test subjects experienced 8.7% more power for 1 kilometer and 8.1% more power for 4 kilometers compared to a control group of noninterval racers.

Research dating as far back as two decades shows that short, intense bursts of exercise zap considerably more bodyfat than sustained activity, even though the interval itself burns mostly glycogen. That's because intervals can ramp up the metabolism and fat-burning for as long as 24 hours afterward. Low-intensity aerobic training doesn't come close.

Even more interesting, there's a link between intervals and human growth hormone (HGH), a muscle-building, fat-stripping chemical produced in the pituitary gland that tells kids' bodies to grow. Since HGH isn't needed much in adulthood, its levels fall, and by age 60 they're just 20% of what they were during the teenage years. Intervals, however, can bring them roaring back for two hours — plenty of time to effect a host of positive changes.

A 2002 study in the *Journal of Sports Sciences* showed that 30 seconds of all-out cycling increased HGH levels by 530% compared to the base levels of non-exercising subjects. The same year, a study in *Sports Medicine* found that both aerobic exercise and strength training stimulate a release of HGH, and that exercising at a greater intensity — as in interval training — stimulates a greater release. In a 2003 study in the *Journal of Clinical Endocrinology & Metabolism*, researchers were left to conclude that "the beneficial effects of exercise can mimic the effects of (artificial) HGH treatment."

More than 500,000 Americans pay up to $1,000 a month for artificial HGH injections, hoping for more muscle; less fat; better recovery, sleep, sexual desire and connective tissue; and thicker, wrinkle-free skin. Getting your HGH boost from exercise won't cost you money, but there is a price.

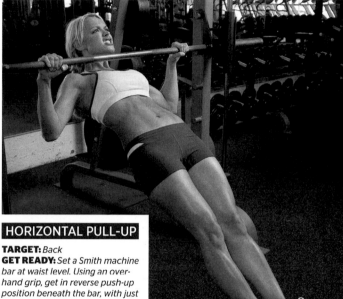

HORIZONTAL PULL-UP

TARGET: *Back*
GET READY: *Set a Smith machine bar at waist level. Using an overhand grip, get in reverse push-up position beneath the bar, with just your heels touching the floor and your body forming a straight line.*
GO: *Arch your back, raise your hips and drive your elbows down to lift your chest to the bar. Squeeze your lats at the top, then slowly return to the start.*

Can You Hack It?

Unfortunately, the intensity that makes these intervals work can't get easier as you get fitter. To keep the HGH benefits package rolling, you must prevent your body from adapting to the stimulus. Otherwise, you'll end up like the cyclists in the New Zealand study: Their performance gains plateaued after 8–12 sessions.

Bottom line, you must constantly push yourself and mix in different activities. It doesn't matter what type of cardio you do — a recumbent bike like Avellina, running stairs or doing "mountain climbers" (push-up position with feet sliding in and out on glider plates) the way Traverso does, or an upright bike and treadmill, which melted the weight off Bryant. Just keep turning up the intensity.

You don't have to start with eight sprints, either. "At first, I'd gas out at four or five," Bryant says. Avellina still isn't at eight sprints, but she has increased the resistance on her recumbent bike from level 8 to 13 for her sprints and from 1 to 3 for her recovery. And as the

Chapter 18

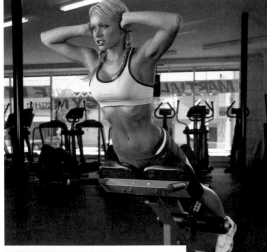

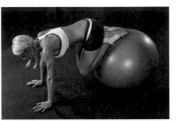

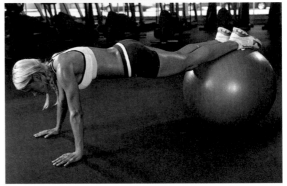

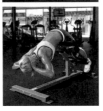

BACK EXTENSION

TARGETS: *Lower back, glutes, hamstrings*
GET READY: *Secure your feet and place your hands lightly on the sides of your head. Keep your back straight and arched, and your eyes forward.*
GO: *Lower your torso by bending at the hips, keeping your back arched and your head in line with your spine. Squeeze your low back, glutes and hamstrings to return to the start position.*

EXERCISE-BALL ROLL-IN

TARGET: *Abs*
GET READY: *Begin in push-up position with your hands shoulder-width apart on the floor, and feet and shins atop an exercise ball.*
GO: *Keeping your back flat, contract your abs and roll your feet forward on the ball to bring your knees toward your chest, then explode backward, pushing the ball back out to the start.*

---

part-time personal trainer decreased her workout time from "45 minutes of drudgery to a few fleeting minutes of crank, crank, crank," she spread the word.

"I have yet to find anyone who loves doing cardio, but they like this," she says. "You can't read a magazine while you do it; you can't even check your heart rate. You have to totally focus on your body and that 30 seconds and getting completely spent. And before you know it, the time flies by and it's over."

Superinterval Tips

➲ **Do any cardio exercise:** run, bike, elliptical, row, swim, jump-rope, etc.
➲ **Don't go all-out on the first interval.** Let your body get used to the higher heart rate. Push harder on interval 2, then let loose on intervals 3–8. Push so hard that you cannot go longer than 30 seconds.
➲ **Vary your use of the machines.** Try the elliptical with and without hands. To ramp up intensity on the treadmill, boost speed or elevation. Use the recumbent bike one day and the upright another. On the upright, alternate intervals standing up and sitting down.
➲ **Never do the same aerobic exercise two days in a row.** Since this is actually a strength workout, your muscles require 48 hours to heal. If you need a daily cardio fix, follow a run day with a swim or bike day.
➲ **If you're new to training,** perform at least three weeks of moderate sprints to strengthen the connective tissue in your joints and prepare your muscles for full-bore exertion.

Superinterval Workouts

Because the superinterval plan is a cardio routine with eight all-out efforts, each designed to cue your body to produce a large spurt of chemicals like HGH, it's technically a strength workout. Still, we've added strength exercises before and after the interval session to complement the cardio without tiring you out. In keeping with the "super" format that floods your body with HGH, these strength moves should also be done all-out. Think of it as a 30-minute total-body cardio/strength "workout sandwich:" five minutes of warm-up strength exercises, 20 minutes of superintervals and five minutes of cool-down strength moves.

Warm-Up Strength Exercises
Duration: 5 minutes

These dynamic multijoint moves are a good warm-up for any aerobic activity because they hit the legs, core and upper body in a coordinated, full-extension manner. They both strengthen and stretch, expanding the lungs and rib cage to prepare for the increased heart rate and respiration you'll experience during intervals. **Note:** The goal here is to warm up, not exhaust yourself. You must be fresh for the sprints to elicit the maximum HGH spurt.

PERFORM FOUR SETS:

15 bodyweight squats

15 exercise-ball roll-ins

15 push-presses with a 10–20-pound weight plate

15 back extensions

Superinterval Workout
Duration: 20 minutes

Start with three minutes at a slow, easy pace, accelerating a bit in minutes 2 and 3. Next comes the first of eight 30-second, all-out, face-twisting, lung-heaving sprints. Follow with 90 seconds at an easy pace to recover for the next sprint. Repeat this pattern seven more times, then finish with a minute of cool-down. Remember, these are general guidelines for a 20-minute workout. If you need more warm-up time or a longer rest interval, take it.

Cool-Down Strength Exercises
Duration: 5 minutes

This workout shouldn't be fun if you pushed hard on the superintervals. It uses squats again (because they're a great lower-body strengthener) but changes the upper-body exercises to complementary push/pull moves not previously addressed.

PERFORM FOUR SETS:

15 bodyweight squats

15 push-ups

15 horizontal pull-ups

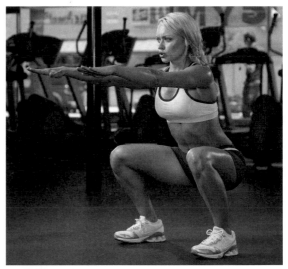

SQUAT

TARGETS: *Quads, hamstrings, glutes*
GET READY: *Stand erect with your feet wider than shoulder width and toes pointing out. Keep your head up, back arched and arms extended in front of you.*
GO: *With your weight entirely on your heels, push your glutes back, and bend your hips and knees as if to sit in a chair until your thighs are past parallel to the floor. Drive through your heels to return to standing.*

PUSH-UP

TARGETS: *Chest, triceps*
GET READY: *Lie facedown on the floor with your hands outside shoulder width, palms and toes touching the floor. Your body should form a straight line. Push up to full-arm extension.*
GO: *Lower your body by bending your elbows until your chin and chest near the floor. Then explode up to the start, keeping your spine arched slightly throughout.*

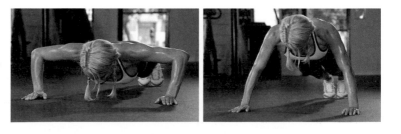

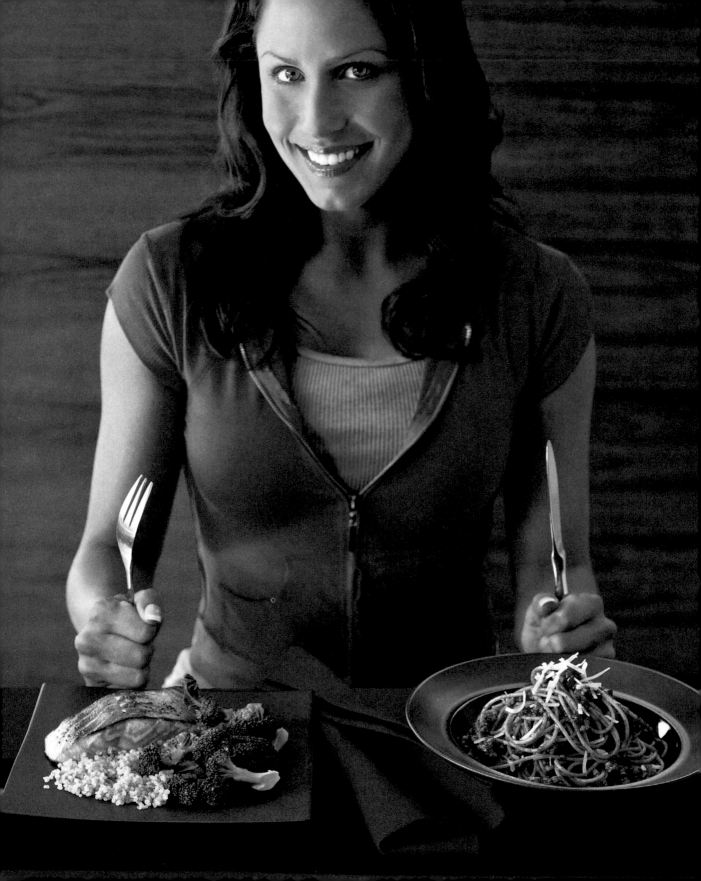

Carb Concepts

Atkins and South Beach took low-carb diets from disparaged to celebrated, but some confusion remains. We clear the air

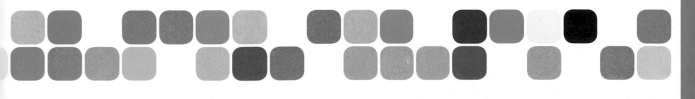

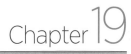

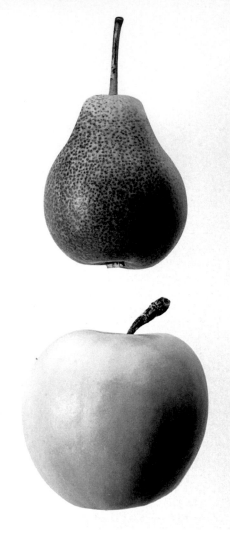

Low-carb diets have had their moment in the spotlight. Is their 15 minutes of fame up? That would be a shame. After all, tons of scientific studies and real-world evidence have shown us that controlling carbs is one of the best ways to manage your weight, keep your heart healthy and increase muscle mass. Many nutritionists, though, don't agree. In the 1970s, the American Medical Association decried low-carb diets (which actually have been popular on and off since the 19th century) as dangerous, and demonized dietary fat as the cause of soaring obesity and heart-disease rates.

In a way, we understand their reasoning. Most of the misconceptions about carbs are based on some type of fact, albeit misinterpreted, misappropriated or just plain mangled. For instance, fat is more than twice as calorie-dense as protein or carbohydrates, containing 9 calories per gram compared to 4 for carbs and protein. Nutritionists used to see it as a simple numbers game, but that was before we understood just how healthy fats can be, how desperately the body needs them, and about the potentially damaging interplay between carbs and insulin within the body. Given all the misconceptions that arise in the mainstream media and our affinity for disseminating the truth about diet and nutrition, we figured we'd do some low-carb myth-busting. Read on to iron out any remaining confusion about following a low-carb lifestyle.

1 Myth: Going low-carb means you can never eat carbs — ever.

This is categorically false. A low-carb diet allows plenty of room for carbs, and M&F HERS encourages you to eat them. We recommend you consume about 1 gram of carbs per pound of bodyweight per day on workout days, dropping to 0.5 gram per pound of bodyweight on rest days. This means that a 140-pound woman can eat 140 grams of carbs on workout days. (To get an idea of just how much food that translates to, see the chart at right.)

The types of carbohydrates you eat and when you eat them are equally important. The majority of the carbs you consume should be slow-digesting, a category that includes foods such as brown rice, legumes, oatmeal, vegetables, whole-wheat bread and, to a certain degree, fruits. The only time we veer from this advice is in the postworkout window. The goal then is to provoke a massive wave of the anabolic hormone insulin to fuel muscle growth and recovery, and to do that you should eat fast-digesting carbs such as jelly, sports drinks, and white bread, potatoes and rice.

Here, then, is an example of what the carb portion of a typical workout day looks like on a low-carb diet:

MEAL	FOOD	CARBS
Breakfast	1 cup oatmeal	25 g
Snack	6 whole-wheat crackers	18 g
Lunch	1 slice whole-wheat bread	13 g
Preworkout	1 large apple	30 g
Postworkout	1 large slice angel food cake	32 g
Dinner	1 cup broccoli	6 g
	1 cup spinach	1 g
		Total: 125 g[1]

[1] Since a 140-pound woman is technically allotted 140 grams of carbs, the remaining 15 grams come from other foods such as peanut butter and cottage cheese. See "Low-Carb, Corrected Diet" on page 139 for a full day's worth of low-carb eating.

2) Myth: By not eating carbs, you'll be hungry all the time.

That's also false. It's true that carbs are the easiest source of energy and eating them increases serotonin levels, a reward system built by evolution to encourage consumption of foods that provide fast, ample energy. But once you adapt to a low-carb diet, your body won't miss them.

Eating carbs may make you feel good, but they won't keep you full for long. Fast-digesting carbs exit the stomach and are absorbed by the intestines quickly; the resulting insulin spike sends glucose to muscle cells, the liver or fat stores, then your body wants more. Protein and fat take longer to process, keeping your digestive system busy — and you satiated — longer.

Protein intake has been shown to reduce hunger by another method as well. A study conducted at University College London had subjects eat three meals: one high in protein, one high in carbs and one high in fat. Scientists found that subjects who consumed the high-protein meal were three times as satiated as after the high-carb meal and twice as satiated as after the high-fat meal. The cause? Peptide YY, a compound produced in the gut after protein consumption that tells the brain you're full. Subjects eating the protein meal had significantly higher levels of peptide YY in their bloodstreams than the others. When low-carb dieters get a greater percentage of calories from protein, they actually experience less hunger than those eating a "normal" higher-carb diet.

3) Myth: You don't have any energy on a low-carb diet.

This myth persists because it contains a minuscule nugget of truth. Glucose is the easiest thing for the body to use as fuel, and all carbs are eventually broken down into glucose. So when you eat ample carbs, your body doesn't have to work very hard to find fuel from other sources, namely fat. Remove or reduce the amount of glucose you provide your body and it'll have to step up fat-burning, which means it must call on special enzymes that break down fat.

The problem is your body is an extremely efficient machine, and it'll slow the production of hormones, enzymes or other compounds that it doesn't currently require in large quantities. When you switch to a low-carb diet, your body may not have an adequate amount of fat-burning enzymes available to break down enough fat to supply all the energy it requires. The result? Sluggishness and lassitude — at least until your body increases its production of fat-burning enzymes.

Ample evidence indicates that this low-energy state is temporary, however, lasting only until the body adapts. A review of research published in 2004 in the journal *Nutrition & Metabolism* states that not only have hunting cultures such as the Inuit survived for thousands of years on low-carb diets out of necessity but "submaximal endurance performance can be sustained despite the virtual exclusion of carbohydrate from the human diet" as well. This is supported by a study conducted by researchers at California State University, Fullerton, who examined the effects of a carb-restricted diet on 15-rep strength in a variety of exercises. They found that a low-carb diet had no effect on the amount of weight subjects could lift.

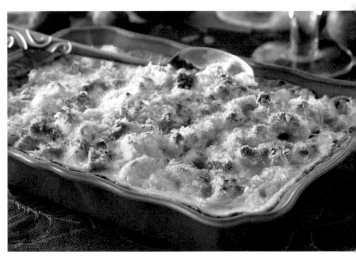

4) Myth: Get ready to gorge yourself on bacon and cheese.

This was Atkins' selling point, but it's just not going to work over the long haul. While low-carb diets do allow for an increase in the number of calories you obtain from fats, your health and physique will be better off if those fats are healthy. You can occasionally indulge in bacon or full-fat cheese, but for the most part aim to eat healthy fat from sources such as avocados, grass-fed beef, olives or olive oil, peanut butter, tuna and wild salmon.

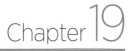
5) Myth: All those fatty foods you're eating now will lead to heart disease.

We've all had the message that fatty foods increase our risk of cardiovascular disease drubbed into us, but research shows saturated fats don't have as much of an effect on health when eaten in place of carbs.

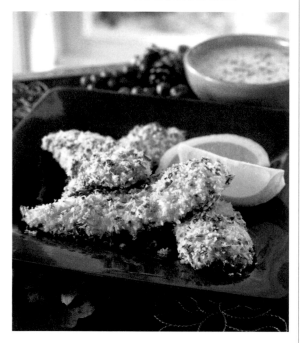

A review of research published in the journal *Nutrition & Metabolism* in 2005 revealed that limiting carbs and replacing them with any type of fat — even the so-called "bad" saturated variety — resulted in both lower triglyceride levels and an increase in "good" HDL cholesterol. In fact, saturated fat elevated HDL cholesterol more than unsaturated fat did. The review also found that the major type of sat fat in beef, chicken and pork doesn't raise "bad" LDL cholesterol levels.

In case you're still worried about eating red meat, other data support its safety. Researchers at the University of Western Australia School of Medicine (Perth) increased subjects' red-meat consumption for eight weeks and compared their markers of oxidative stress and inflammation, two signals of heart disease, to those who maintained their normal diets. No difference was seen in the markers but subjects who ate more red meat had lower levels of C-reactive protein, a powerful inflammatory factor that's closely linked to heart disease. It appears, then, that replacing at least some carb calories with fat can make you healthier.

6) Myth: Following a low-carbohydrate diet will cause you to lose muscle.

This myth has traceable roots as well, though they've been twisted by misconception. When you first begin a low-carb diet, you'll lose a little of the water stored in muscle tissue, making your muscles look slightly less full. This is because fewer dietary carbs are circulating and the fat-burning pathway isn't yet fully operational, so your body will use the glycogen stored in muscles as fuel. Glycogen normally pulls water into muscle cells, so with reduced glycogen levels, you also get reduced water levels. As your system adapts, however, it'll restore glycogen levels and your muscle volume will return to its previous state. At no time will you lose actual muscle tissue; in fact, following a low-carb diet will help boost muscle growth while you get lean, primarily because you're taking in more protein, which spurs protein synthesis and burns more fat for fuel.

A study published in a 2002 issue of the journal *Metabolism* showed the power of a low-carb diet and its effects on body composition. Scientists at the University of Connecticut (Storrs) had 12 men switch to a very low-carb diet. At the end of six weeks, subjects had experienced significant decreases in bodyfat and an increase in lean body mass, despite the fact they hadn't trained. You read that right: Eating a low-carb diet can actually increase muscle mass even if weightlifting isn't involved.

7) Myth: Low-carb diets are a short-term solution.

Here's the bottom line: If you follow our dietary advice, you're most likely already on a relatively lower-carb diet. It's very difficult to eat clean and improve your physique while still consuming massive amounts of chips and cookies. Those of you who eat clean and love to train already know this way of eating isn't a quick fix, it's a lifestyle. Once you commit to it, you'll experience all the benefits we've discussed: healthier arteries, increased strength and muscle mass, and a leaner physique. And that's no myth.

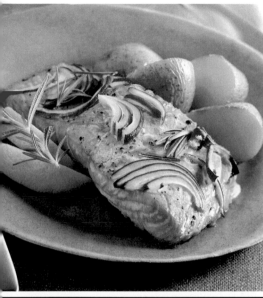

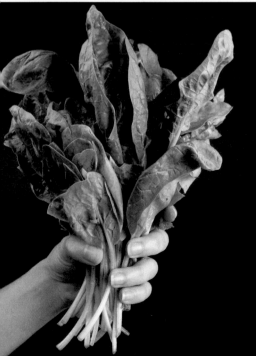

Low-Carb, Corrected Diet

	CALORIES	PROTEIN (G)	CARBS (G)	FAT (G)
BREAKFAST				
2 large whole eggs	148	12	1	10
2 large egg whites	34	8	0	0
1 cup oatmeal	147	6	25	2
SNACK				
2 Tbsp. peanut butter	188	8	6	16
6 whole-wheat crackers	108	2	18	4
LUNCH				
3 oz. deli turkey breast	94	21	0	1
1 slice whole-wheat bread	70	2	13	1
1 cup lettuce	10	1	2	0
1 Tbsp. light mayo	50	0	1	5
PREWORKOUT				
1 scoop whey protein	85	20	1	0
1 large apple	110	0	30	0
POSTWORKOUT				
1 scoop whey protein	85	20	1	0
1 large slice angel food cake (one-sixth of cake)	144	3	32	0
DINNER				
6 oz. salmon	312	34	0	18
1 cup broccoli	31	3	6	0
1 cup raw spinach	7	1	1	0
1 Tbsp. olive oil/ vinegar dressing	72	0	0	8
BEFORE-BED SNACK				
1 cup low-fat cottage cheese	163	28	6	2
TOTALS:	**1,858**	**169**	**143**	**67**

NOTE: Mix all protein powders according to directions on label.

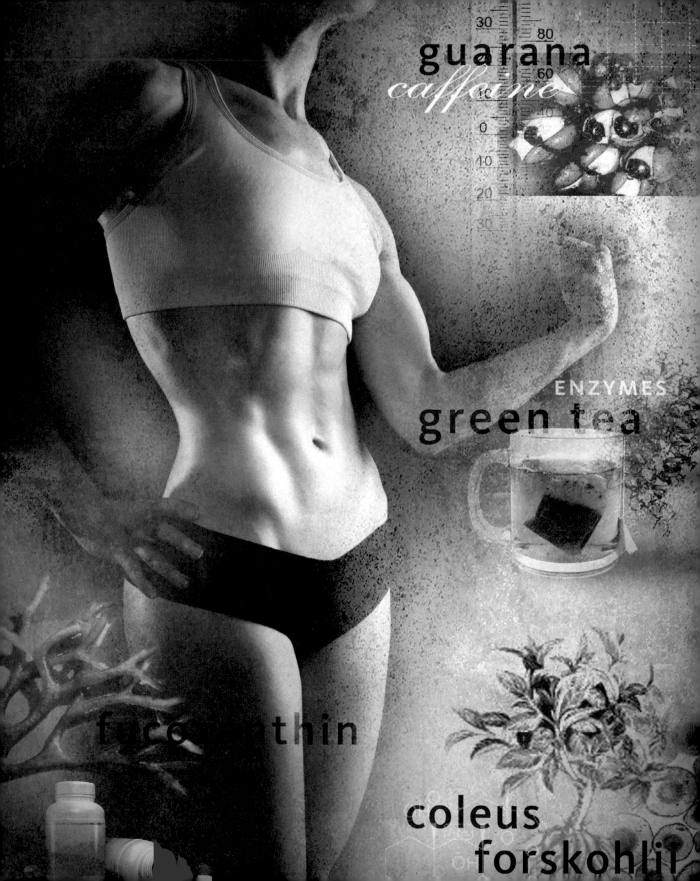

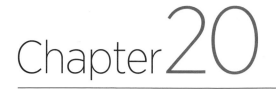

Chapter 20

Farewell to Fat

If your efforts to lean out have hit a wall, ignite your metabolic blowtorch with these natural fat-fighters

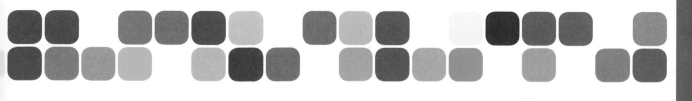

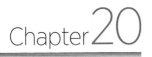

Your latest weight-loss effort started off fast but has recently sputtered and slowed. It seems like the fat is clinging tighter than a preteen to her Robert Pattinson poster. The truth is, getting lean isn't easy. You often have to deal with lethargy, hunger and frustrating stagnation to the point where it feels like your own body is working against you. Unfortunately, that's a pretty accurate description.

Your body has evolved into being great at self-preservation, which means not only storing new fat but also keeping the fat you already have on your frame.

When you restrict calories, your metabolism ultimately slows down to preserve its remaining energy stores. It's as if your body is fighting every step of the way in a misguided attempt to survive. But if you can head off the signals that shut down fat loss before they take hold, you can ensure your fat-burning efforts get a green light all the way to your destination.

If you want to regain metabolic control, consider the following all-natural ingredients for showing your fat stores who's really in charge, just before you burn them off.

Guarana

The botanical guarana is a favorite of native cultures across the globe for its energy-boosting properties. A main component of this plant is caffeine, which is an even more potent fat-burner than you might think. In fact, caffeine alone has several benefits that warrant a second look.

The most noticeable effect of any supplement is a thermogenic property, and guarana is no exception. This means it ramps up the body's metabolic rate to burn more calories, which often results in a perceptible increase in body temperature. Another predominant effect known as lipolysis refers to the breakdown of bodyfat. Among the various weight-loss effects, this one is more intuitive because the stored fat must be broken down before it can be burned as energy.

Speaking of energy consumption, this works hand in hand with the aforementioned thermogenic effect. It's exactly what you need: the one-two punch of fat breakdown and subsequent fat-burning. Research published in *The American Journal of Clinical Nutrition* showed that caffeine consumption alone increased lipolysis and fired up metabolic rate to the point that caloric expenditure was elevated 13%.

Guarana offers additional fat-burning benefits, including the ability to train more frequently through the amelioration of muscle soreness. "When training for fat loss, the more work you can get done, the more calories you can burn," says Mike T. Nelson, CSCS, a PhD candidate at the University of Minnesota (Minneapolis). "Unfortunately, hard training can induce muscle soreness, making your return trip to the gym less than fun. Caffeine can reduce this transient pain, allowing you to train harder the next time and ensuring that you keep burning those calories." Not only that, but caffeine can increase the total amount of work you do in each session, which burns more calories, he adds.

➔ **Dose:** 200–600 mg as needed for energy, enhanced mental focus and fat loss.

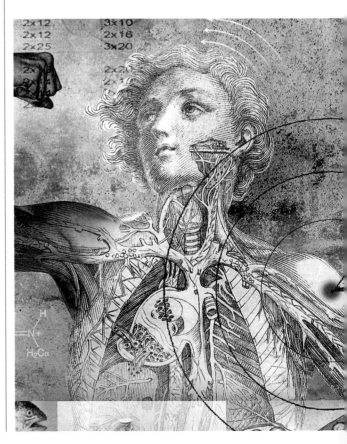

Green Tea

Not to be outdone, green tea throws its hat into the thermogenic ring. While this less-processed version of black tea does contain caffeine, its thermogenic properties also come courtesy of substances known as catechins. Green tea contains epigallocatechin gallate (EGCG), which has exciting health-boosting and fat-burning effects. It encourages thermogenesis by indirectly affecting the way in which hormones attack fat stores.

Normally, in an attempt to keep a death grip on metabolism, your body will fight fat loss by quickly hindering the work of enzymes that initiate the process of burning stored energy. EGCG attacks one of these inhibitory enzymes responsible for clamping down on hormonally stimulated fat-burning. By blocking the inhibitor, this catechin acts like a bouncer at a club, keeping the troublemakers away from the thermogenic event. This ensures your fat-fighting furnaces are stoked and running at full power.

One reason green tea and EGCG work so well is they're not alone in their quest to reduce bodyfat. Caffeine contributes to this process, and they work cooperatively to provide an even more potent thermogenic stimulus. Specifically, green tea and caffeine together disrupt undesirable enzyme activity from phosphodiesterase (PDE), which is all too good at shutting down the fat-loss powerplant. Blocking the effect of PDE allows fat loss to continue unabated and increases the thermogenic effect. In support of these concepts, a study in the journal *Obesity* confirmed that drinking catechin-rich green tea, without exercise or other diet intervention, can reduce both waist size and bodyfat levels.

➲ **Dose:** Drinking green tea is a great idea, but you should also take about 500 mg of green tea extract standardized for EGCG three times daily before meals. Research shows the catechins from the extract are better absorbed than from the tea.

Coleus Forskohlii

You'll want to consider a third component to the green tea-and-caffeine cocktail: an extract from a tropical plant called coleus forskohlii known as forskolin. This substance works on the other end of fat-fighting enzymes: Rather than preventing inhibitors from blocking fat loss, forskolin actually stimulates those that start the fire.

Activating fat-loss enzymes is likely the most conventional method for igniting lipolysis, which is one reason forskolin is growing in popularity. It doesn't bother with inhibiting the inhibitors; it increases levels of the cellular messenger known as cAMP and essentially flips the "on" switch for fat loss. Because other natural fat-fighters ensure this switch stays on, the result is a powerful fat-loss combination. A 2005 study conducted at the University of Kansas (Lawrence) showed that after 12 weeks of forskolin supplementation, bodyfat percentage decreased while bone mass increased in obese subjects.

➲ **Dose:** Take a coleus forskohlii supplement standardized for 20–50 mg forskolin 2–3 times daily before meals.

Fucoxanthin

Did you know there are two types of bodyfat and that one of them, brown fat, is paradoxically responsible for the function of fat-burning? Unfortunately, we don't have much of this helpful adipose as adults, but a newer supplement may trick the body into thinking it does.

Dubbed fucoxanthin, this seaweed-derived ingredient may turn on genes in regular white adipose — the kind you're trying to lose — that resemble those of brown fat. In particular, this supplement increases levels of a thermogenic protein called UCP-1 that optimizes the way energy is expended. But fucoxanthin also appears to turn off the genes involved in white fat cell growth and development. Not only is more energy burned, but additional fat growth may be inhibited. Theory aside, preliminary animal research from Hokkaido University (Hakodate, Japan) shows that the combination of these effects is enough to induce weight loss.

➲ **Dose:** Early availability of supplemental fucoxanthin suggests a daily total of 15 mg in divided doses. For enhanced absorption, take it with your daily fish-oil capsule or after a fat-containing meal.

Turkey & Egg White Wrap

SERVES 2

- ½ Tbsp. olive oil
- ½ lb. ground turkey
- ½ tsp. ground cumin
- 6 egg whites
- Kosher salt
- Cracked black pepper
- 1 medium tomato, diced
- ¼ cup chopped cilantro
- 2 whole-wheat tortillas

NUTRITION FACTS (per serving):
359 calories
32 g protein
29 g carbs
14 g fat
5 g fiber
1 g sugar
550 mg sodium

1 / Heat olive oil in a medium nonstick skillet, then add turkey and cumin. Crumble turkey as it cooks to a light golden brown, then add egg whites.

2 / Continue stirring until eggs are completely white. Season with salt and pepper to taste. Add tomato and cilantro, stir for one minute and remove from heat.

3 / In a separate skillet, warm tortillas until soft. Divide turkey-egg mixture evenly into tortillas, roll like a burrito and serve immediately.

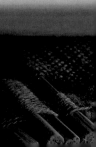

Break *the Fast*

The most important meal of the day doesn't have to be the most boring one

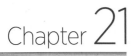

For many of us, there isn't a feeling more pleasant than awaking to the faint clatter of pans and spatulas, and the smell of coffee brewing. Yet those halcyon mornings seem like a dream when you face the reality of getting kids to school, making time for the gym or adjusting your schedule to avoid traffic on the way to work.

This wouldn't be the first time you've heard that eating breakfast is important. After all, the first meal of the day is crucial for replenishing energy levels and feeding your hungry muscles, which have gone without fuel for close to 10 hours.

These are simple and healthy ways to start your day right. They not only provide enough quality protein and healthy fats to keep you satisfied for hours but are also fast and tasty, and set you up to eat smart the rest of the day.

Strawberry & Basil Smoothie

SERVES 2

- 2 cups fresh or frozen strawberries
- Zest from half a lemon
- 1 scoop plain or vanilla whey protein powder
- 1 cup ice
- ½ cup water
- 1 cup plain Greek yogurt
- 2 basil leaves

NUTRITION FACTS (per serving):
223 calories
32 g protein
20 g carbs
2.5 g fat
8 g fiber
5 g sugar
118 mg sodium

1 / Purée all ingredients in a blender until smooth. Serve immediately. Garnish with a dollop of yogurt and basil if desired.

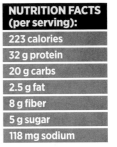

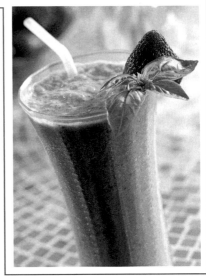

Steamed Asparagus & Fried Eggs

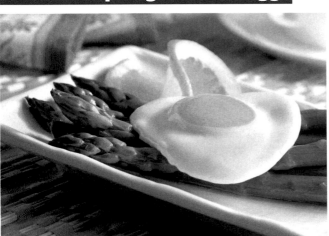

SERVES 1

- 14 asparagus spears
- 1 Tbsp. olive oil, divided
- Kosher salt
- Cracked black pepper
- 2 eggs

NUTRITION FACTS
230 calories
18 g protein
10 g carbs
14 g fat
4 g fiber
0 g sugar
251 mg sodium

1 / Place asparagus in a steamer basket in a large saucepan with 1 inch of water. Bring to a boil, reduce heat and steam for 3–4 minutes until asparagus is bright green. Season with 1 teaspoon olive oil, salt and pepper. Remove from heat and cover to keep warm.

2 / Coat a small nonstick skillet with remaining olive oil and place over medium heat. Crack eggs into skillet, and season with salt and pepper. When egg whites are cooked, flip them and remove from heat.

3 / Let eggs sit for one minute, then serve atop asparagus. When the yolks are popped it will create a dressing for the asparagus.

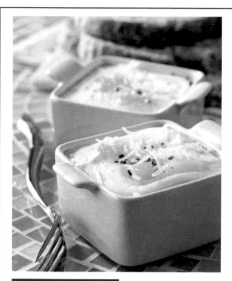

Baked Eggs With Parmesan

SERVES 1
- 2 eggs
- Kosher salt
- Cracked black pepper
- Parmesan cheese, grated

1 / Preheat oven to 400 degrees F. Meanwhile, crack eggs into a 4-ounce oven-safe ramekin. Sprinkle liberally with salt and pepper. Place ramekin in a baking dish, then add hot water around the ramekin until it reaches the level of the eggs.

2 / Bake for 20 minutes or until eggs are cooked to your liking.

3 / Sprinkle liberally with Parmesan cheese. Serve with whole-wheat toast or fruit.

NUTRITION FACTS (eggs only):
214 calories
18 g protein
2 g carbs
14 g fat
0 g fiber
0 g sugar
545 mg sodium

Caramelized Onion, Roasted Red Pepper & Broccoli Frittata

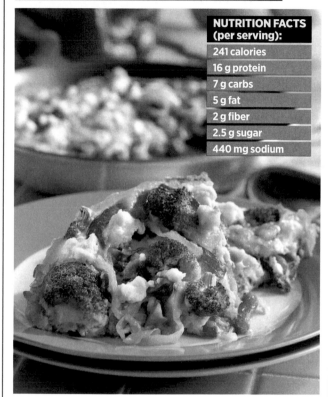

NUTRITION FACTS (per serving):
241 calories
16 g protein
7 g carbs
5 g fat
2 g fiber
2.5 g sugar
440 mg sodium

SERVES 2
- ½ Tbsp. olive oil
- ½ onion, sliced thin
- 1 egg
- 4 egg whites
- Salt and pepper
- ½ red bell pepper, roasted, seeded and sliced thin
- ½ cup broccoli florets
- 1 tsp. chopped thyme
- 1 Tbsp. goat cheese

1 / Preheat oven to 350 degrees F. Heat olive oil in a medium nonstick, ovenproof skillet over low heat. Add onion and cook until golden brown.

2 / In a medium bowl, whisk egg, egg whites, salt and pepper.

3 / Add red bell pepper, broccoli and thyme to skillet. Increase heat to medium and toss for two minutes until broccoli is bright green. Stir in eggs and crumble goat cheese on top.

4 / Reduce heat to low for two minutes, then place skillet in oven. (Wrap handle in foil if it's not ovenproof.) Bake until light golden brown and puffed up, 10–12 minutes. Cut into wedges.

Salmon Soba

SERVES 1

- 2 oz. soba noodles*
- 1 Tbsp. olive oil
- 1 Tbsp. lemon juice
- 2 tsp. rice wine vinegar
- ¼ tsp. wasabi paste*
- 1 pouch (6 oz.) pink salmon
- 1 Tbsp. roasted sesame seeds*

* found in the Asian aisle of your supermarket

1 / Prepare soba according to package directions. Meanwhile, whisk together olive oil and lemon juice in a small bowl.

2 / Add vinegar and wasabi, whisking until smooth. Combine all ingredients in a large bowl.

NUTRITION FACTS

551 calories
51 g protein
44 g carbs
21.5 g fat

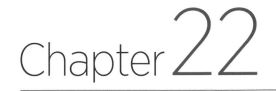

Chapter 22

Cool Protein

You should know by now how cool we think protein is, but this chapter offers recipes for protein dishes served cold

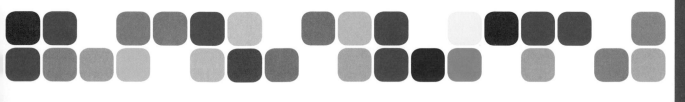

Chapter 22

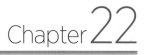

There's a time when a hot meal can't be beat. But when the only place you can bear to sweat is at the gym, not over a hot stove, try these cold protein meals.

Technically, last night's leftovers qualify as cold protein, and anyone can grill a steak and then chill it for later, but in reality those foods are meant to be eaten warm. These recipes, on the other hand, are best served cold, straight from the icebox. While a few of them do need several minutes of stovetop time, they can also be made ahead and — you guessed it — stored in the fridge.

Thai Beef Salad

SERVES 1

- 2 cups torn romaine lettuce pieces
- 1/4 medium red onion, thinly sliced
- 1/4 cucumber, peeled, seeded and sliced
- 1 medium tomato, cut into eighths
- 6 oz. sliced deli roast beef, cut in strips
- 1 Tbsp. soy sauce
- 2 Tbsp. lime juice
- 1/2 tsp. brown sugar
- 2 tsp. water

1/ Arrange first five ingredients on a plate or in a bowl. In a separate small bowl, whisk soy sauce and lime juice together.

2/ Add brown sugar and water, whisk until smooth and pour over salad.

NUTRITION FACTS

332 calories

36 g protein

20 g carbs

12 g fat

Tuna-Stuffed Peppers

SERVES 1

- 1 Tbsp. light mayo
- 1 tsp. Dijon mustard
- 2 tsp. apple cider vinegar
- 1 can (6 oz.) white albacore tuna in water, drained
- 1/2 cup cole slaw mix
- 1 red (or yellow or orange) bell pepper, cut in half and seeded

1 / In a medium bowl, mix mayo and mustard until blended.

2 / Add vinegar and stir well. Add tuna and mash together with a fork.

3 / Stir in cole slaw, then divide mixture between pepper halves.

NUTRITION FACTS

321 calories
42.5 g protein
10 g carbs
10 g fat

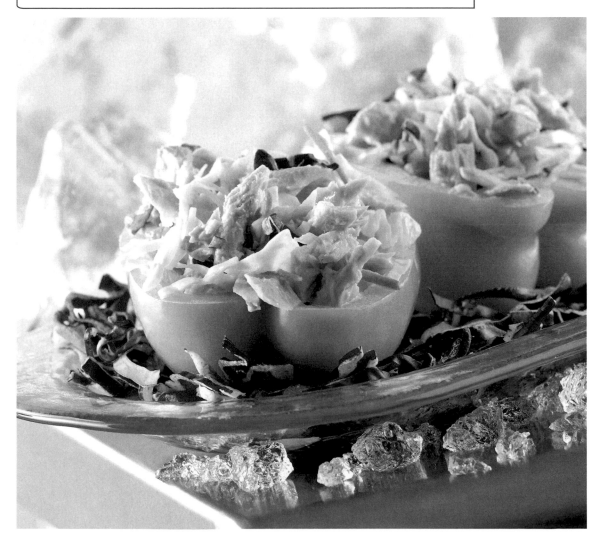

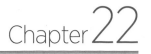

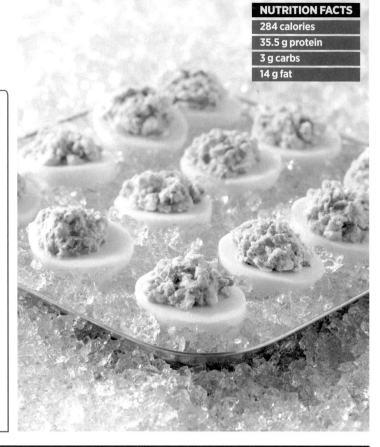

NUTRITION FACTS

284 calories
35.5 g protein
3 g carbs
14 g fat

Spicy Deviled Eggs

SERVES 1

- 6 eggs
- 2 Tbsp. low-fat cottage cheese
- Salt to taste
- Hot sauce to taste
- 1 green onion, thinly sliced

1 / Place eggs in a large saucepan, fill with hot water and bring to a boil. Remove from heat, cover and allow to cook for about 10 minutes.

2 / Transfer pan to sink and run eggs under cold water. When cooled, peel eggs and cut them in half lengthwise.

3 / Carefully remove yolks, discarding three of them. Place remaining yolks in a small bowl with cottage cheese. Mash with a fork until smooth, then add salt and hot sauce to taste. Spoon yolk mixture into egg white halves and top with green onion.

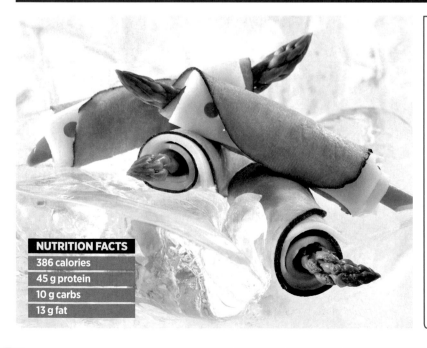

NUTRITION FACTS

386 calories
45 g protein
10 g carbs
13 g fat

Ham Roll-Ups

SERVES 1

- 4 oz. sliced low-fat deli ham
- 4 oz. sliced low-fat Swiss cheese (like Jarlsberg Lite)
- 1 Tbsp. light mayo
- 4 asparagus spears

1 / Place one slice of ham on a flat work surface, top with one slice of cheese and spread with a little light mayo.

2 / Place an asparagus spear at one end (perpendicular to the ham/cheese) and roll up. Repeat with remaining ingredients.

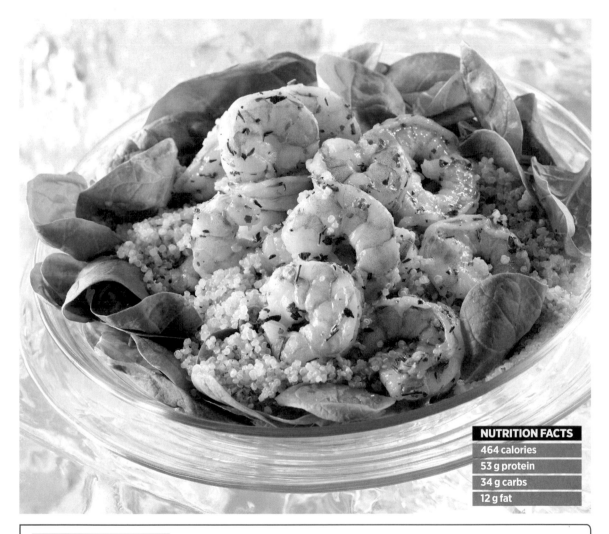

NUTRITION FACTS

464 calories
53 g protein
34 g carbs
12 g fat

Shrimp Quinoa Spinach Salad

SERVES 1

- 8 oz. shrimp, precooked and frozen
- Garlic salt
- Italian seasoning
- 1/2 cup water
- 1/4 cup dry quinoa
- 1 Tbsp. red wine vinegar
- 1 tsp. olive oil
- 2 cups fresh spinach leaves

Note: This dish requires extra time to season and defrost the shrimp. If you didn't plan ahead, skip the seasonings and just place the shrimp in a colander under cold running water to defrost more quickly.

1 / Place shrimp in a zip-top plastic bag and sprinkle liberally with garlic salt and Italian seasoning. Close bag tightly and shake gently to spread spices throughout; lay flat in the refrigerator for two hours or until shrimp has thawed.

2 / Meanwhile, bring water and quinoa to a boil in a small saucepan over high heat. Reduce heat to low, cover and simmer, stirring occasionally, until all water is absorbed, about seven minutes. Let cool.

3 / In a small bowl, whisk together vinegar and olive oil.

4 / Arrange spinach on a plate, spread quinoa over the top, then add shrimp and dressing.

● Orzo is made from semolina flour, a fairly fast-digesting carbohydrate that can get to muscle fibers quickly for better recovery. That makes this salad a good accompaniment to your postworkout protein shake.

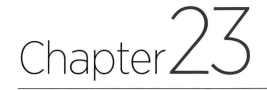

Chapter 23

Salad Days

*We just made the perfect summer
meal a delicious all-year favorite*

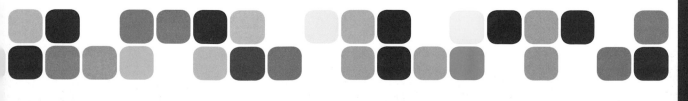

Do you want a meal that's light and cool, but which also nourishes and satisfies? You need a kick-ass salad.

These salads aren't the penitent combination of iceberg lettuce and bottled dressing that you watched your mom suffer through when you were growing up. These are true meals, each boasting a generous helping of protein, a smart mix of antioxidant- and fiber-rich fruits and vegetables, and satisfying healthy fats to ensure you're not hungry an hour later.

In fact, there's a salad here for any kind of eating plan and any time of day. They're quick and easy, and made with simple ingredients. Get ready to add five new meals to your regular rotation.

NUTRITION FACTS (per serving):

274 calories	
26 g protein	
1 g carbs	
19 g fat	
1 g fiber	
0 g sugar	
161 mg sodium	

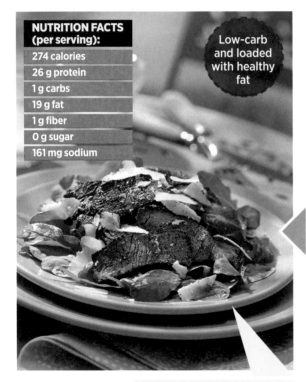

Low-carb and loaded with healthy fat

● Olive oil is rich in healthy monounsaturated fat, which enhances heart health and is preferentially burned during exercise instead of stored as bodyfat. Olive oil also contains the phytonutrient oleocanthal for joint recovery.

Seared Tuna Salad With Green Beans, Red Bell Pepper, Olives & Orzo *(previous page)*

SERVES 2

- 8 oz. Grade A tuna, cut into a square or triangle, not steaks
- 1 Tbsp. cumin
- Kosher salt and cracked black pepper
- ½ tsp. extra-virgin olive oil
- ½ cup thinly sliced green beans (sliced across)
- ½ cup thinly sliced roasted red bell pepper
- ½ oz. olives, kalamata or nicoise
- 1 cup cooked orzo pasta
- ¼ tsp. dried oregano
- 2 tsp. red wine vinegar
- 4 cups baby spinach

NUTRITION FACTS (per serving):

390 calories	
34 g protein	
48 g carbs	
9 g fat	
6 g fiber	
5 g sugar	
348 mg sodium	

1 / Season tuna with cumin, salt and pepper. Heat a sauté pan or skillet to high heat, then add olive oil.

2 / Carefully place tuna in pan and brown all sides; the center should stay bright pink and the gray should be no more than ¼-inch thick. Let cool, then slice thinly.

3 / Toss remaining ingredients, and season with salt and pepper.

4 / Place salad on a serving plate and arrange tuna on top. Serve immediately.

Steak Salad With Arugula, Lemon, Olive Oil & Parmesan

SERVES 2

- 8 oz. filet mignon, sliced in half
- Kosher salt and cracked black pepper
- 4 small handfuls arugula
- Juice of one lemon
- 1 Tbsp. extra-virgin olive oil
- ¼ cup grated or 1 oz. shaved Parmesan cheese
- Nonstick cooking spray

1 / Heat a grill to high heat and lightly coat it with nonstick cooking spray. Season steak with salt and pepper, and grill to desired doneness.

2 / Toss arugula with lemon juice and olive oil, and season with salt and pepper. Slice steak and place it on top of salad.

3 / Garnish with Parmesan cheese. Serve immediately.

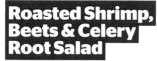

Roasted Shrimp, Beets & Celery Root Salad

SERVES 2

- 8 shrimp (about ½ pound), cleaned
- Kosher salt and cracked black pepper
- 1 tsp. extra-virgin olive oil
- 3 beets, red or yellow, tops removed
- 1 celery-root bulb
- 1 Tbsp. light mayo
- Juice of one lemon
- Bitter greens such as arugula, mizuna or radicchio

1/ Preheat oven to 400 degrees F. Lightly season shrimp with salt and pepper, and toss with olive oil.

2/ Arrange shrimp on a baking sheet, place in oven and cook until light pink, about 5–10 minutes. (You could do this a day ahead.)

3/ In a large saucepan, cover beets with water and bring to a boil, cooking until they're fork-tender. Cooking time will vary depending on the beets' size.

4/ Remove from heat and place beets in ice water to cool. Their skin should peel easily by rubbing.

5/ Cut peeled beets into small wedges, and season with salt, pepper and a dash of olive oil. (You could do this up to two days ahead.)

6/ Cut both ends off celery root, then cut off remaining skin. Slice thinly into matchsticks. Toss with mayo and lemon juice. (You could do this a day ahead.)

7/ On a serving plate, place celery-root mixture in a large strip. Place beets on top. Line up shrimp on top of beets. Toss bitter greens with a dash of olive oil and garnish salad with a few leaves. Serve immediately.

● *Beets are a good source of betaine, which not only enhances liver and joint repair but has also been shown to increase strength and power.*

NUTRITION FACTS
(per serving):

184 calories	
25 g protein	
14 g carbs	
3 g fat	
3 g fiber	
8 g sugar	
559 mg sodium	

Low-calorie!

Grilled Tofu Salad With Cabbage, Cucumber, Carrot & Rice Wine Vinaigrette

SERVES 2

- 4 large slices firm tofu
- 1 Tbsp. rice wine vinegar
- 2 tsp. peanut butter
- 1 Tbsp. chopped ginger
- 2 tsp. low-sodium soy sauce
- 3 Tbsp. extra-virgin olive oil
- 1 cup shredded red cabbage
- 1 cup shredded Savoy or Napa cabbage
- ½ cup thinly sliced cucumber matchsticks
- ½ cup thinly sliced carrot matchsticks
- Nonstick cooking spray

1 / Heat a grill to high heat. Coat tofu with nonstick cooking spray and carefully lay it on grill, turning to a 90-degree angle to make grill marks. Repeat on the other side. Let cool, then slice thinly.

2 / Whisk together rice wine vinegar, peanut butter, ginger and soy sauce. While whisking, slowly pour in olive oil. (This will make extra dressing.)

3 / Toss remaining ingredients with tofu and 1–2 tablespoons of dressing. Serve immediately.

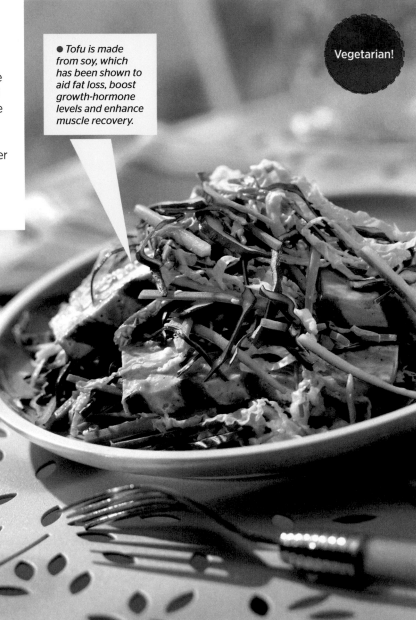

● *Tofu is made from soy, which has been shown to aid fat loss, boost growth-hormone levels and enhance muscle recovery.*

Vegetarian!

NUTRITION FACTS (per serving):

320 calories	
41 g protein	
24 g carbs	
29 g fat	
9 g fiber	
5 g sugar	
92 mg sodium	

Spinach Salad With Kale, Strawberries & Grilled Chicken

SERVES 2

- 1 Tbsp. balsamic vinegar
- 1 Tbsp. honey
- 1 garlic clove
- 4 basil leaves
- 2 Tbsp. water
- 2 Tbsp. extra-virgin olive oil
- Kosher salt and cracked black pepper
- 2 cups baby spinach
- 1 cup purple kale leaves
- 1 cup sliced strawberries
- 8 oz. grilled chicken, sliced very thin

1 / In a blender purée vinegar, honey, garlic, basil and water.

2 / While puréeing, slowly add olive oil, salt and pepper. (This will make extra dressing.)

3 / Toss spinach, kale, strawberries and chicken with 1–2 tablespoons of dressing. Serve immediately.

NUTRITION FACTS (per serving):
244 calories
30 g protein
18 g carbs
7 g fat
4 g fiber
8 g sugar
128 mg sodium

Well-balanced and great anytime

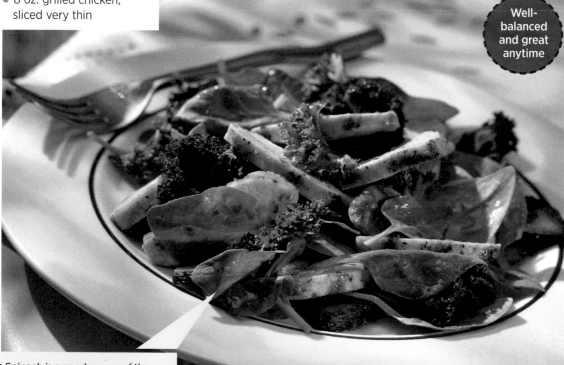

● *Spinach is a good source of the critical amino acid glutamine. It also contains beta-ecdysterone, a phytochemical that enhances muscle recovery, and octacosanol, which has been shown to boost strength.*

BLEND

- ½ cup frozen mixed berries (blueberries, raspberries, strawberries)
- 1 packet instant regular oatmeal
- 1 scoop strawberry whey protein isolate
- ½ cup fat-free vanilla yogurt
- ½–1 cup water

TIP: For a change of pace, swap the oatmeal for shredded wheat bran. It's an excellent source of whole grain and fiber, and a great slow-burning carb.

Whey Isolate

Whey protein isolate contains more protein, and less fat and lactose per serving than regular whey. It breaks down fast and releases amino acids into the bloodstream. That's why we always recommend it when your muscles are most desperate for protein, like first thing in the morning. Plus, research shows that whey reduces hunger so you eat less throughout the day, making fat loss easier.

Fat-Free Yogurt

Besides the obvious health-boosting benefits of protein and calcium, this dairy food does your body good in other ways. It contains more calcium than milk, and has been found to help maximize fat loss — especially around the waistline — and minimize muscle loss. Yogurt is also a good source of glutamine, an important amino acid that helps you lose fat.

Mixed Berries

Red berries like raspberries are extremely fibrous, low in calories and chock-full of bone-building vitamin K. The pectin found in blackberries helps keep blood-sugar levels on an even keel. Blueberries are great for shedding fat because they contain pterostilbene, a compound that helps the body break down fat and cholesterol.

Oatmeal

The carbs in oatmeal are slow-digesting and won't boost insulin levels, which means you'll stay energized longer without interfering with fat-burning.

Shake It Up

Try these four recipes for a refreshing twist on your protein shakes

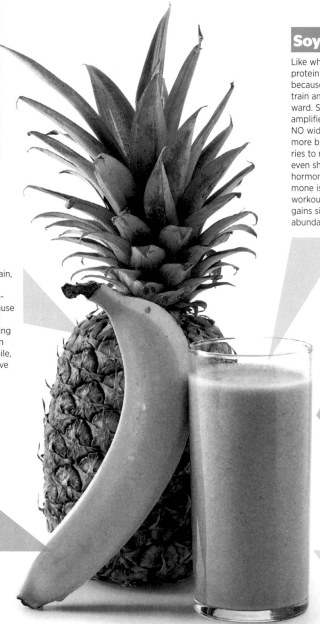

PIÑA COLADA PUNCH

WHEN: Preworkout

NUTRITION FACTS: 260 calories, 28 g protein, 32 g carbs, 4 g fat

BLEND

1   small banana

¼   cup chopped pineapple

1   cup unsweetened vanilla almond milk

½   scoop vanilla whey protein isolate

½   scoop vanilla soy protein isolate

    Ice

Soy Isolate

Like whey, soy is a fast-digesting protein that's ideal around workouts because it gives you more energy to train and enhances recovery afterward. Studies also show that soy amplifies nitric-oxide (NO) levels. NO widens blood vessels, allowing more blood and the nutrients it carries to reach your muscles. Research even shows that soy boosts growth-hormone levels. This anabolic hormone is critical for women around workouts to boost size and strength gains since testosterone isn't in abundant supply.

Pineapple

Pineapple contains bromelain, a proteolytic enzyme that helps your body digest protein. This is important because it can prevent bloating and indigestion before and during your workout, and assists in protein utilization. Meanwhile, the potassium will help stave off muscle cramps.

Whey Isolate

Intense workouts wreak havoc on your muscles, and they need protein to heal and grow. Whey isolate is the fastest way to get a heap of protein to your muscle fibers, and drinking it preworkout ensures it's there when your muscles need it for energy and to prevent breakdown.

Banana

Bananas are an ideal preworkout fruit because they contain fructose and glucose to give both an instant and sustained energy boost. (Fructose is low-glycemic, which the body consumes slowly.) They're also easy to digest, and full of potassium and vitamin C, which are vital for proper muscle function. Plus, potassium can boost your metabolism.

Almond Milk

Almonds usually make the list of nature's healthiest foods, and for good reason: They're rich in magnesium, manganese, selenium, and vitamins D and E. Almond milk is also low in fat and lactose-free, making it a great alternative to cow's milk.

CHOCOLATE-APPLE CRUNCH

WHEN: Morning or Preworkout

NUTRITION FACTS: 380 calories, 35 g protein, 55 g carbs, 3 g fat

Whey Isolate

Topping off your morning shake with whey protein isolate is the quickest way to replenish muscle protein and fend off catabolism. Used preworkout, it provides amino acids to build muscle.

Apple

Aside from being a good slow-digesting carb, apples are full of antioxidants. They also contain polyphenols, which have been found to increase endurance and strength and even promote fat loss, especially around the midsection.

Granola

For all its popularity, granola may be one of the most controversial breakfast foods. The cereal is made from rolled oats and nuts, and is coated with honey. Rolled oats provide fiber, which enhances digestion, and honey provides carbs to restock glycogen levels. So the sugar gives you an instant lift and the complex carbs provide sustained energy.

BLEND

- ½ cup chopped frozen apple
- ½ cup low-fat granola
- 1 scoop chocolate whey protein isolate
- 1 cup water
- Ice

TIP: Preworkout, consider replacing half the whey with soy protein isolate.

AVOCADO AVALANCHE

WHEN: Bedtime

NUTRITION FACTS: 273 calories, 26 g protein, 9 g carbs, 16 g fat

BLEND

- 1½ ripe avocados
- 1 scoop vanilla casein protein powder
- 1 packet Splenda (optional)
- Ice

Casein Protein

Casein is an excellent source of high-quality protein. Because it digests slower than whey, studies show it minimizes the body's tendency to ravage your muscles for fuel while you sleep.

Avocado

The fat in avocados is primarily the healthy monounsaturated variety, which is less likely to be stored as bodyfat. Avocados also contain mannoheptulose, a sugar that actually blunts insulin release (to keep fat storage at bay and fat-burning turned up) and enhances calcium absorption.

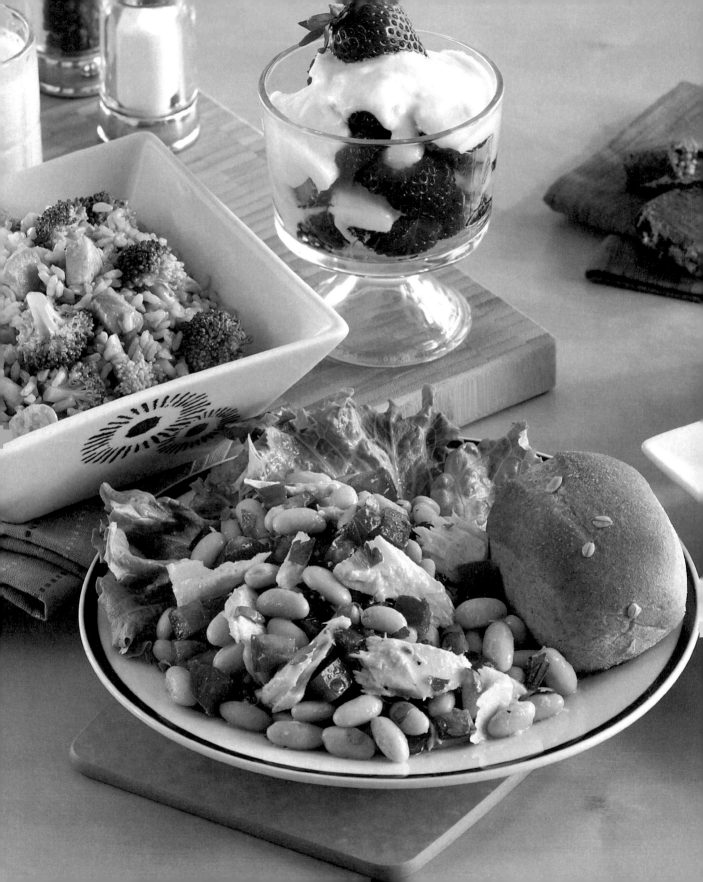

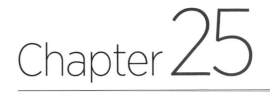

The No-Sweat Diet

Get rid of those last stubborn pounds with this easy-prep, two-week meal plan. Repeat until you reach your goal weight

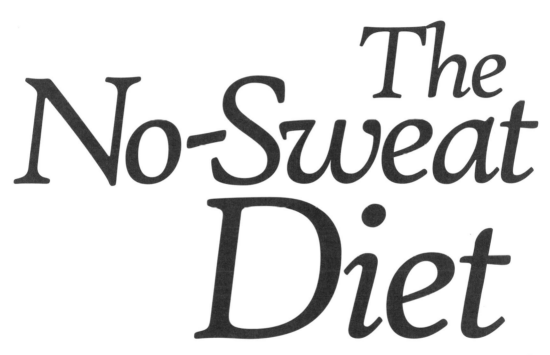

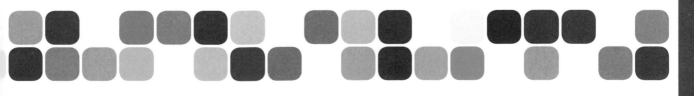

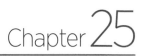
WEEK 1

SUNDAY DAY 1

BREAKFAST
1 whole-grain waffle
topped with
  1 Tbsp. natural peanut butter
  1 medium banana, sliced
8 oz. 1% milk
1 cup coffee

LUNCH
Tuna-White Bean Salad:
  1 cup canned white beans,
    drained
  3 oz. canned light tuna,
    drained
  1 small tomato, chopped
  1 Tbsp. Italian dressing
1 whole-wheat dinner roll

PREWORKOUT SNACK
Iced latte (6 oz. coffee and
  6 oz. 1% milk over ice)
1 meal replacement bar
  (40/30/30, about
  200 calories)
(or 15 g whey protein powder
  [¾ scoop] mixed with water)

POSTWORKOUT SNACK
1 cup low-fat plain yogurt
topped with
  1 cup sliced strawberries
  1 Tbsp. sunflower seeds
(or 30 g whey protein powder
  [1½ scoops] mixed with water)

DINNER
Chicken Stir-Fry:
  5 oz. boneless, skinless
    chicken breast and
  ½ cup sliced onion,
    sautéed in 2 tsp. peanut oil
  1 Tbsp. low-sodium
    soy sauce
  1 Tbsp. rice wine vinegar
1 cup steamed broccoli
1 cup cooked brown rice

DAILY TOTALS:
1,874 calories, 129 g protein,
251 g carbs, 54 g fat (24%),
35 g fiber

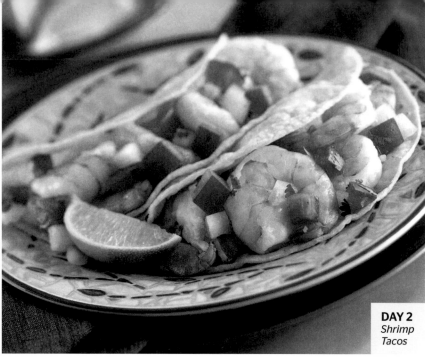

DAY 2
Shrimp Tacos

MONDAY DAY 2

BREAKFAST
1 cup cooked oatmeal
topped with
  ¼ cup raisins
  1 tsp. brown sugar
8 oz. 1% milk
1 cup coffee

LUNCH
Curried Egg Salad Sandwich:
  1 hard-boiled egg and
  4 hard-boiled egg whites,
    chopped
  1 Tbsp. light mayo
  1 tsp. yellow curry powder
  1 whole-wheat pita
8 oz. calcium- and vitamin D-
  fortified orange juice

PREWORKOUT SNACK
¼ cup roasted soy nuts
1 medium pear
(or 15 g whey protein powder
mixed with water)

POSTWORKOUT SNACK
2 cinnamon graham crackers
  each topped with
    3 Tbsp. fat-free ricotta cheese
15 grapes
(or 30 g whey protein powder
mixed with water)

DINNER
Shrimp Tacos:
  2 6-inch corn tortillas
  20 large shrimp, sautéed
    in 2 tsp. olive oil
  ¾ cup canned black beans,
    drained
  ¼ cup chopped onion
  ½ cup diced tomato
  1 Tbsp. lime juice

DAILY TOTALS:
1,860 calories, 106 g protein,
271 g carbs, 42 g fat (20%),
33 g fiber

TUESDAY DAY 3

BREAKFAST
1 cup high-fiber ready-to-eat
  cereal (at least 4 g fiber/cup)
1 cup raspberries
1 Tbsp. chopped nuts
  (walnuts/almonds/pecans)
8 oz. 1% milk
1 cup coffee

LUNCH
Veggie Burger:
  Veggie patty (such as
    Gardenburger or
    Boca Burger)
  1 whole-grain bun
  Sliced onion and tomato

  1 oz. reduced-fat
    cheddar cheese
  1 Tbsp. ketchup or mustard
1 cup pineapple chunks

PREWORKOUT SNACK
½ Turkey Sandwich:
  1 slice whole-wheat bread
  2 oz. sliced deli turkey breast
  1 Tbsp. light mayo
(or 15 g whey protein powder
mixed with water)

POSTWORKOUT SNACK
Smoothie:
  blend until frothy
  4 oz. 1% milk
  4 oz. calcium- and vitamin D-
    fortified orange juice
  ½ cup fat-free vanilla yogurt
  ½ cup frozen strawberries
  1 Tbsp. protein powder
(or 30 g whey protein powder
mixed with water)

DINNER
5 oz. roasted/broiled pork
  tenderloin
1 medium baked sweet potato
2 cups spinach, sautéed in
  2 tsp. olive oil
1 whole-grain dinner roll

DAILY TOTALS:
1,865 calories, 117 g protein,
242 g carbs, 55 g fat (26%),
38 g fiber

WEDNESDAY DAY 4

BREAKFAST
Fruit and Yogurt Parfait:
   1 cup low-fat plain yogurt
   1 medium banana, sliced
   2 Tbsp. low-fat granola
   1 Tbsp. chopped nuts
      (walnuts/almonds/pecans)
1 cup coffee

LUNCH
Chicken Caesar Wrap:
   1 whole-wheat tortilla
   4 oz. roasted boneless,
      skinless chicken breast
   1 cup chopped romaine
      lettuce
   2 Tbsp. light Caesar dressing
   1 Tbsp. grated
      Parmesan cheese
1 cup watermelon chunks

PREWORKOUT SNACK
1 apricot
1 oz. almonds (about 22)
(or 15 g whey protein powder
mixed with water)

POSTWORKOUT SNACK
8 oz. 1% milk
2 Fig Newtons
(or 30 g whey protein powder
mixed with water)

DINNER
Fennel Orange Salad:
   1 orange, peeled and sliced
   ¼ cup sliced fennel
   ¼ cup sliced onion
   Balsamic vinegar to taste

Scallops Marinara:
   5 oz. scallops, sautéed in
      1 tsp. olive oil
   1½ cups cooked spaghetti
   ¾ cup marinara sauce

DAILY TOTALS:
**1,845 calories, 105 g protein,
246 g carbs, 52 g fat (25%),
21 g fiber**

THURSDAY DAY 5

BREAKFAST
1 whole-grain waffle
   topped with
   1 Tbsp. natural peanut butter
   1 medium banana, sliced
8 oz. 1% milk
1 cup coffee

LUNCH
1 cup salad greens
   1 Tbsp. Italian dressing
Pita Pizza:
   1 whole-wheat pita
   broil after topping with
   ½ cup marinara sauce
   ¼ cup shredded part-skim
      mozzarella cheese
   ½ cup thawed,
      frozen spinach

PREWORKOUT SNACK
Iced latte (6 oz. coffee and
   6 oz. 1% milk over ice)
1 meal replacement bar
   (40/30/30, about
   200 calories)
(or 15 g whey protein powder
mixed with water)

POSTWORKOUT SNACK
½ cup vanilla frozen yogurt
   topped with
   ½ cup blackberries
(or 30 g whey protein powder
mixed with water)

DINNER
1 cup black bean soup
5 oz. grilled/broiled
   tuna steak
6 steamed asparagus spears
1 cup cooked brown rice

DAILY TOTALS:
**1,868 calories, 122 g protein,
254 g carbs, 46 g fat (22%),
31 g fiber**

FRIDAY DAY 6

BREAKFAST
1 cup cooked oatmeal
   topped with
   ¼ cup raisins
   1 tsp. brown sugar
   1 Tbsp. chopped nuts
      (walnuts/almonds/pecans)
8 oz. 1% milk
1 cup coffee

LUNCH
1 cup chili
   topped with
   ¼ cup shredded low-fat
      cheddar cheese
6-inch corn tortilla
1 cup pineapple chunks

PREWORKOUT SNACK
1 medium apple
½ cup roasted soy nuts
(or 15 g whey protein powder
mixed with water)

POSTWORKOUT SNACK
½ cup fat-free ricotta cheese
   topped with
   ½ cup dried fruit
      (raisins/cherries/
      cranberries/apricots)
(or 30 g whey protein powder
mixed with water)

DINNER
Turkey Scaloppine:
   5 oz. pounded turkey breast
      and 1 garlic clove, chopped,
      sautéed in 1 tsp. olive oil

1 Tbsp. fresh lemon juice
1 Tbsp. capers
1 cup cooked couscous
1 cup steamed green beans

DAILY TOTALS:
**1,892 calories, 110 g protein,
256 g carbs, 54 g fat (25%),
34 g fiber**

SATURDAY DAY 7

BREAKFAST
4 4-inch pancakes
   topped with
   4 Tbsp. light maple syrup
   1 cup sliced strawberries
2 turkey sausage links
1 cup coffee

LUNCH
Tuna Sandwich:
   3 oz. canned light tuna,
      drained
   1 Tbsp. light mayo
   5 grapes, halved
   1 Tbsp. chopped walnuts
   2 slices whole-wheat bread
8 oz. calcium- and vitamin D-
   fortified orange juice

PREWORKOUT SNACK
1 cup steamed edamame
(or 15 g whey protein powder
mixed with water)

POSTWORKOUT SNACK
1 piece part-skim string cheese
1 medium pear
(or 30 g whey protein powder
mixed with water)

DINNER
Grilled Chicken Sandwich:
   5 oz. grilled chicken breast
   Sliced onion and tomato
   1 Tbsp. mustard
   1 whole-wheat bun
Cucumber Salad:
   1 cucumber, sliced
   1 Tbsp. rice wine vinegar
   1 tsp. sesame or canola oil

DAILY TOTALS:
**1,850 calories, 120 g protein,
227 g carbs, 52 g fat (25%),
29 g fiber**

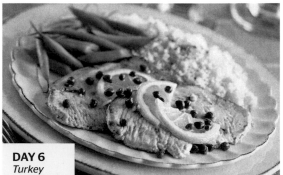

DAY 6
*Turkey
Scaloppine*

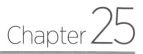
WEEK 2

SUNDAY DAY 8

BREAKFAST
Egg Sandwich:
  2 poached eggs
  1 whole-wheat English muffin
  1 slice fat-free
    American cheese
8 oz. calcium- and vitamin D-
  fortified orange juice
1 cup coffee

LUNCH
Turkey Sandwich:
  3 oz. sliced deli turkey breast
  2 slices whole-wheat bread
  2 Tbsp. cranberry sauce
  1 lettuce leaf
1 cup cantaloupe chunks

PREWORKOUT SNACK
¼ cup hummus
10 baby carrots
(or 15 g whey protein powder
mixed with water)

POSTWORKOUT SNACK
8 oz. 1% milk
2 Fig Newtons
(or 30 g whey protein powder
mixed with water)

DINNER
5 oz. broiled lean flank steak
1 medium baked potato
2 Tbsp. light sour cream
2 cups spinach, sautéed in
  1 tsp. olive oil
½ cup fat-free frozen yogurt
  topped with
  1 cup raspberries

DAILY TOTALS:
**1,858 calories, 113 g protein,
249 g carbs, 50 g fat (24%),
29 g fiber**

MONDAY DAY 9

BREAKFAST
1 cup high-fiber ready-to-eat
  cereal (at least 4 g fiber/cup)
1 cup blueberries
1 Tbsp. chopped nuts
  (walnuts/almonds/pecans)
8 oz. 1% milk
1 cup coffee

LUNCH
Ham Sandwich:
  3 oz. lean deli ham
  1 Kaiser roll
  1 oz. reduced-fat
    cheddar cheese
  1 lettuce leaf and tomato slice
  1 Tbsp. honey mustard
6 oz. low-sodium
  vegetable juice

PREWORKOUT SNACK
½ medium banana, sliced
  dipped in
  1 Tbsp. dark chocolate chips,
    melted in microwave
8 oz. 1% milk
(or 15 g whey protein powder
mixed with water)

POSTWORKOUT SNACK
Trail Mix:
  ¼ cup roasted soy nuts
  2 Tbsp. raisins
  1 Tbsp. sunflower seeds
(or 30 g whey protein powder
mixed with water)

DINNER
1 cup vegetable soup
5 oz. broiled salmon
1 cup cooked brown rice
1 cup steamed broccoli

DAILY TOTALS:
**1,853 calories, 113 g protein,
250 g carbs, 53 g fat (25%),
30 g fiber**

TUESDAY DAY 10

BREAKFAST
1 cup cooked oatmeal
  topped with
  ¼ cup raisins
  1 tsp. brown sugar
  1 Tbsp. chopped nuts
    (walnuts/almonds/pecans)
8 oz. 1% milk
1 cup coffee

LUNCH
10 shrimp
  1 Tbsp. cocktail sauce
Veggie Burger:
  Veggie patty (such as
    Gardenburger or
    Boca Burger)
  1 whole-grain bun

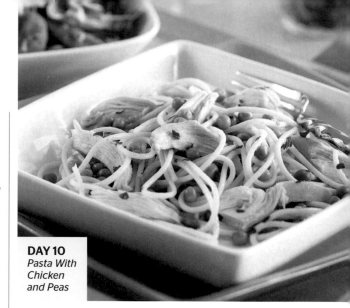

DAY 10
*Pasta With
Chicken
and Peas*

Sliced onion and tomato
  1 oz. reduced-fat
    cheddar cheese
  1 Tbsp. ketchup or mustard

PREWORKOUT SNACK
1 granola bar (100 calories)
8 oz. 1% milk
(or 15 g whey protein powder
mixed with water)

POSTWORKOUT SNACK
Smoothie:
  blend until frothy
  4 oz. 1% milk
  4 oz. calcium- and vitamin D-
    fortified orange juice
  ½ cup fat-free vanilla yogurt
  ½ cup frozen strawberries
  1 Tbsp. protein powder
(or 30 g whey protein powder
mixed with water)

DINNER
Pasta With Chicken and Peas:
  1½ cups cooked spaghetti
  ½ cup marinara sauce
  ¼ cup peas
  3 oz. roasted chicken breast
Spinach Salad:
  1 cup baby spinach
  1 Tbsp. Italian dressing
  1 Tbsp. grated
    Parmesan cheese

DAILY TOTALS:
**1,853 calories, 120 g protein,
245 g carbs, 44 g fat (21%),
24 g fiber**

WEDNESDAY DAY 11

BREAKFAST
Fruit and Yogurt Parfait:
  1 cup low-fat plain yogurt
  1 medium banana, sliced
  2 Tbsp. low-fat granola
  1 Tbsp. chopped nuts
    (walnuts/almonds/pecans)
1 slice whole-wheat toast with
  2 tsp. natural peanut butter
1 cup coffee

LUNCH
Tuna-White Bean Salad:
  1 cup canned white beans,
    drained
  3 oz. canned light tuna,
    drained
  1 small tomato, chopped
  1 Tbsp. Italian dressing
1 whole-wheat dinner roll

PREWORKOUT SNACK
1 medium apple
1 piece part-skim string cheese
(or 15 g whey protein powder
mixed with water)

POSTWORKOUT SNACK
¼ cup hummus
10 baby carrots
(or 30 g whey protein powder
mixed with water)

DINNER
Turkey "Sloppy Joe":
  5 oz. ground white-meat
    turkey, sautéed in 2 tsp.
    olive oil
  1 tsp. taco seasoning
  1 whole-wheat bun

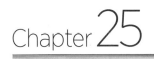

1 ear corn
½ cup fat-free frozen yogurt
topped with
1 cup blackberries

DAILY TOTALS:
**1,810 calories, 114 g protein,
263 g carbs, 49 g fat (22%),
39 g fiber**

THURSDAY DAY 12

BREAKFAST
1 whole-grain waffle
topped with
1 Tbsp. natural peanut butter
1 medium apple, sliced
8 oz. 1% milk
1 cup coffee

LUNCH
Chicken Caesar Wrap:
1 whole-wheat tortilla
4 oz. roasted boneless,
skinless chicken breast
1 cup chopped
romaine lettuce
2 Tbsp. light Caesar dressing
1 Tbsp. grated
Parmesan cheese
1 cup pineapple chunks

PREWORKOUT SNACK
1 medium banana
8 oz. 1% milk
(or 15 g whey protein powder
mixed with water)

POSTWORKOUT SNACK
½ Turkey Sandwich:
1 slice whole-wheat bread
2 oz. sliced deli turkey breast
1 Tbsp. mustard
(or 30 g whey protein powder
mixed with water)

DINNER
Spaghetti and Meatballs:
1½ cups cooked spaghetti
¾ cup marinara sauce
3 meatballs
1 zucchini, sliced, sautéed in
1 tsp. olive oil

DAILY TOTALS:
**1,858 calories, 110 g protein,
242 g carbs, 53 g fat (25%),
27 g fiber**

FRIDAY DAY 13

BREAKFAST
1 cup high-fiber ready-to-eat
cereal (at least 4 g fiber/cup)
1 peach, sliced
1 Tbsp. chopped nuts
(walnuts/almonds/pecans)
8 oz. 1% milk
1 cup coffee

LUNCH
Curried Egg Salad Sandwich:
1 hard-boiled egg and
4 hard-boiled egg whites,
chopped
1 Tbsp. light mayo
1 tsp. yellow curry powder
1 whole-wheat pita
8 oz. calcium- and vitamin D-
fortified orange juice

PREWORKOUT SNACK
2 apricots
1 cup low-fat plain yogurt
(or 15 g whey protein powder
mixed with water)

POSTWORKOUT SNACK
1 meal replacement bar
(40/30/30, about
200 calories)
¼ cup dried fruit (raisins/
cherries/cranberries)
(or 30 g whey protein powder
mixed with water)

DINNER
Turkey Burger:
5 oz. ground white-meat
turkey breast patty,
sautéed in 2 tsp. canola oil
1 whole-wheat bun
Sliced onion and tomato
1 oz. reduced-fat
cheddar cheese
1 Tbsp. steak sauce
1 ear corn
15 grapes

DAILY TOTALS:
**1,888 calories, 113 g protein,
271 g carbs, 52 g fat (23%),
26 g fiber**

SATURDAY DAY 14

BREAKFAST
Egg Sandwich:
2 poached eggs
1 whole-wheat English muffin
1 slice fat-free
American cheese
1 cup coffee

LUNCH
Turkey Sandwich:
3 oz. sliced deli turkey breast
2 slices whole-wheat bread
2 Tbsp. cranberry sauce
1 lettuce leaf
8 oz. calcium- and vitamin D-
fortified orange juice

PREWORKOUT SNACK
2 kiwis
½ cup roasted soy nuts
(or 15 g whey protein powder
mixed with water)

POSTWORKOUT SNACK
2 cinnamon graham crackers
each topped with
3 Tbsp. fat-free ricotta cheese
(or 30 g whey protein powder
mixed with water)

DINNER
5 oz. roasted lean leg of lamb
1 cup peas
1 medium baked sweet potato
2 Tbsp. semisweet or dark
chocolate chips

DAILY TOTALS:
**1,851 calories, 122 g protein,
237 g carbs, 50 g fat (24%),
32 g fiber**

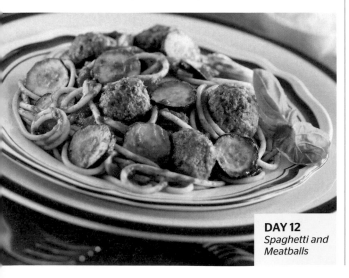

DAY 12
*Spaghetti and
Meatballs*

The Energy Equation

➲ The meals in this plan are based on the needs of
a highly active 145-pound woman and adjusted for
a weekly weight loss of 1½ pounds. Any more than
2 pounds per week may affect muscle mass.

➲ If you weigh less than 145 pounds, subtract a serving
of fruit (50–100 calories), whole-wheat bread (70 calories per 1-ounce slice) or low-fat milk (100 calories per
8 ounces) as needed.

The Top 200 Healthy Muscle Foods
USE THIS CHART TO BUILD YOUR SHOPPING LIST AND DAILY DIET PLANS

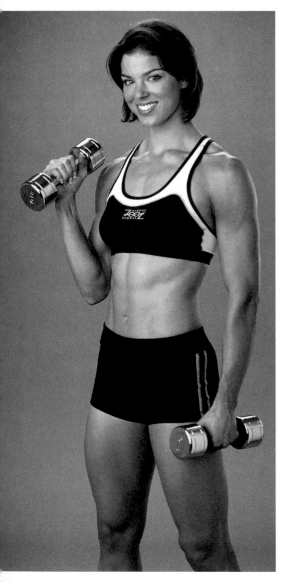

MEAT & EGGS

	CALORIES	PROTEIN*	CARBS*	FAT*
BEEF[1]				
8 oz. beefalo (composite of cuts)	328	56	0	11
8 oz. beef brisket	352	48	0	17
1 oz. beef jerky	116	9	3	7
8 oz. beef liver	312	48	0	8
3 beef ribs, large	474	34	0	37
8 oz. corned beef	448	32	0	34
8 oz. flank steak	352	48	0	16
4 oz. ground beef, 95% lean	152	24	0	6
4 oz. ground beef, 90% lean	196	24	0	11
4 oz. ground beef, 85% lean	240	20	0	17
4 oz. ground beef, 80% lean	284	20	0	22
4 oz. ground beef, 75% lean	328	16	0	28
4 oz. ground beef, 70% lean	372	16	0	34
8 oz. porterhouse steak	560	43	0	42
4 oz. roast beef	106	14	1	5
8 oz. T-bone steak	496	44	0	35
8 oz. tenderloin	560	48	0	25
8 oz. top sirloin	456	48	0	29
8 oz. tri-tip	372	47	0	19
EGGS[1]				
1 egg white, large	17	4	0	0
1 whole egg, large	74	6	0	5
1 whole egg, extra-large	85	7	0	6
1 whole egg, jumbo	96	8	0	6
LAMB[1]				
4 oz. ground lamb	320	20	0	27
8 oz. lamb chops	472	40	0	32
8 oz. leg of lamb	472	40	0	32
PORK[1]				
1 rack baby-back ribs (roasted)	810	53	0	65
3 slices bacon	311	8	0	31
8 oz. cured ham	464	48	0	30
4 oz. ground pork	300	20	0	24
1 Italian sausage	391	16	1	35
1 pork chop, large	205	20	0	13
8 oz. pork tenderloin	312	48	0	12
4 oz. smoked deli ham	186	21	1	11
1 link smoked sausage	265	15	1	22

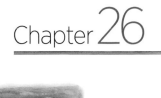

	CALORIES	PROTEIN*	CARBS*	FAT*
POULTRY[1]				
6 oz. chicken breast	185	39	0	2
4 oz. chicken breast deli meat	95	21	0	1
1 chicken thigh	82	14	0	3
6 chicken wings (Buffalo wings)	366	34	6	22
1 Cornish game hen (roasted)	295	51	0	9
6 oz. duck, domesticated	226	31	0	10
4 oz. ground ostrich	188	23	0	10
4 oz. ground turkey	170	20	0	9
6 oz. turkey breast	189	42	0	1
4 oz. turkey deli meat	104	22	2	0
1 oz. turkey jerky	101	19	1	1
SEAFOOD[1]				
1 Alaskan king crab leg	144	31	0	1
6 oz. bass	194	32	0	6
6 oz. catfish	230	26	0	13
6 clams, medium	66	11	2	1
6 oz. cod	140	30	0	1
1 crab cake	160	11	5	10
1 Dungeness crab	140	28	1	2
3 oz. eel (mixed species)	156	16	0	10
6 oz. flounder	154	32	0	2
6 oz. haddock	148	32	0	1
6 oz. halibut	188	36	0	4
1 lobster, medium	135	28	1	1
6 oz. mackerel (mixed species)	268	34	0	13
6 mussels, medium	84	11	4	2
6 oysters, medium	57	6	3	2
6 oz. salmon (Atlantic)	312	34	0	18
1 can sardines (in oil, drained)	191	23	0	11
6 oz. scallops	150	28	0	2
6 oz. sea bass	164	32	0	3
4 oz. shrimp	120	23	1	2
6 oz. sole	154	32	0	2
3 oz. squid (fried calamari)	149	15	7	6
6 oz. swordfish	206	34	0	7
6 oz. trout	252	36	0	11
1 can light tuna (in water)	191	42	0	1
1 can white tuna (in water)	220	41	0	5
6 oz. whitefish	228	32	0	10

* values in grams   [1] Raw unless otherwise noted.   [2] Cooked unless otherwise noted.

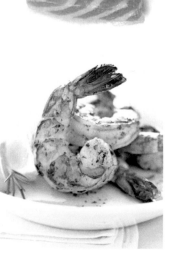

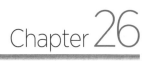
DAIRY

	CALORIES	PROTEIN*	CARBS*	FAT*
CHEESE				
1 slice low-fat American cheese	38	5	1	1
1 slice cheddar cheese	113	7	0	9
8 oz. low-fat cottage cheese (1%)	163	28	6	2
8 oz. cottage cheese (small curd)	232	28	6	10
1 slice low-fat Monterey Jack cheese	88	8	0	6
1 oz. part-skim mozzarella cheese	72	7	1	5
1 slice provolone cheese	98	7	1	7
1 slice low-fat Swiss cheese	50	8	1	1
MILK/MILK PRODUCTS				
8 oz. fat-free milk	83	8	12	0
8 oz. low-fat milk (1%)	102	8	12	2
8 oz. reduced-fat milk (2%)	122	8	11	5
8 oz. whole milk (3.25%)	146	8	11	8
1 Tbsp. fat-free sour cream	11	0	2	0
1 Tbsp. reduced-fat sour cream	20	0	1	2
YOGURT				
8 oz. fat-free yogurt (fruit)	213	10	43	0
8 oz. low-fat yogurt (fruit)	225	9	42	3
8 oz. low-fat yogurt (plain)	143	12	16	4

FRUITS, JUICES & VEGETABLES

FRUITS				
1 apple, large	110	0	30	0
1 avocado	289	3	15	27
1 banana, medium	105	1	27	0
1 cup blueberries	83	1	21	0
1 cantaloupe, medium	188	5	45	1
½ grapefruit, large	53	1	13	0
1 nectarine, medium	60	1	14	0
1 orange, large	86	2	22	0
1 peach, medium	38	1	9	0
1 pear, medium	96	1	26	0
1 cup sliced pineapple	79	1	20	0
1 cup raspberries	64	1	15	1
1 cup whole strawberries	46	1	11	0
JUICES				
8 oz. apple juice (unsweetened)	117	0	29	0
8 oz. grapefruit juice	96	1	23	0
8 oz. orange juice	110	2	25	1
8 oz. tomato juice	41	2	10	0

* values in grams   ¹ Raw unless otherwise noted.   ² Cooked unless otherwise noted.

	CALORIES	PROTEIN*	CARBS*	FAT*
VEGETABLES				
20 asparagus spears	60	6	12	0
1 cup chopped broccoli	31	3	6	0
1 cup Brussels sprouts	38	3	8	0
1 carrot, medium	25	1	6	0
1 cup chopped cauliflower	28	1	3	0
1 celery stalk, medium	6	0	1	0
1 cup canned corn	133	4	30	2
1 cup eggplant	20	1	5	0
1 can green beans	52	3	12	0
1 onion, medium	46	1	11	0
1 cup peas	118	8	21	1
1 baked potato, medium	161	4	37	0
2 cups salad (greens)	44	3	8	0
1 sweet potato, medium	103	2	24	0
1 tomato, medium	22	1	5	0
½ cup tomato sauce (marinara)	92	2	14	3
1 cup sliced zucchini	29	1	7	0

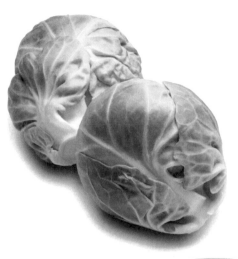

GRAINS
BREAD/CRACKERS

	CALORIES	PROTEIN*	CARBS*	FAT*
1 bagel, medium (plain)	289	11	56	2
1 bran muffin, medium	305	8	55	8
1 dinner roll (plain)	84	2	14	2
1 English muffin (plain)	134	4	26	1
1 English muffin (whole wheat)	134	6	27	1
1 hamburger bun (plain)	120	4	21	2
1 slice multigrain bread	65	3	12	1
1 pita bread (wheat), large	170	6	35	2
1 pita bread (white), large	165	5	33	1
1 slice pumpernickel bread	65	2	12	1
1 slice rye bread	83	3	15	1
6 saltine crackers	154	3	26	4
1 slice white bread	66	2	13	1
1 slice whole-wheat bread	70	3	13	1
6 whole-wheat crackers	108	2	18	4

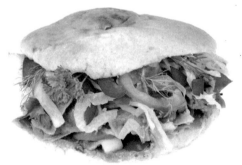

CEREAL

	CALORIES	PROTEIN*	CARBS*	FAT*
1 cup Cheerios	111	4	22	2
1 cup corn flakes	101	2	24	0
1 cup corn grits, cooked	143	3	31	0
1 packet Cream of Wheat (instant)	102	3	22	0
½ cup Grape-Nuts	208	6	47	1
1 cup oatmeal, cooked	147	6	25	2
1 cup Raisin Bran	178	5	43	1
1 cup Rice Krispies	108	2	24	0
1 cup Special K	117	7	22	0
1 cup Wheaties	106	3	24	1

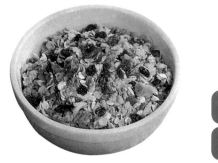

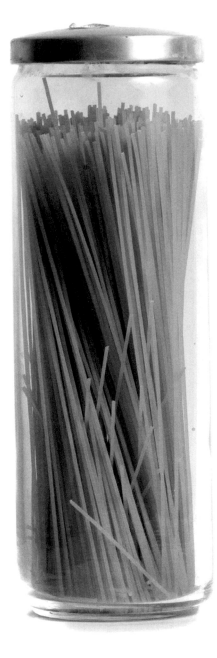

	CALORIES	PROTEIN*	CARBS*	FAT*
PASTA [2]				
1 cup couscous	176	6	36	0
1 cup egg noodles	221	7	40	3
1 cup macaroni and cheese	370	16	68	4
1 cup rice noodles	192	2	44	0
1 cup soba	113	6	24	0
1 cup spaghetti	221	8	43	1
1 cup whole-wheat pasta	174	7	37	1
RICE [2]				
1 cup brown rice (medium grain)	218	5	46	2
1 rice cake	35	1	7	0
1 cup white rice (long grain)	205	4	45	0
1 cup white rice (medium grain)	242	4	53	0
1 cup wild rice	166	7	35	1

LEGUMES & NUTS

LEGUMES [2]				
1 cup baked beans	239	12	54	1
1 cup black beans	227	15	41	1
1 cup chickpeas	286	12	54	3
1 cup edamame (soybeans)	254	22	20	12
½ cup hummus	207	10	18	12
1 cup kidney beans	225	15	40	1
1 cup lima beans	216	15	39	1
1 cup navy beans	255	15	47	1
1 Tbsp. peanut butter	94	4	3	8
1 oz. peanuts	166	7	6	14
1 cup pinto beans	245	15	45	1
1 cup refried beans	237	14	39	3
NUTS				
1 oz. almonds	169	6	5	15
1 oz. cashews	163	4	9	13
1 oz. hazelnuts	183	4	5	18
1 oz. macadamia nuts	203	2	4	22
1 oz. mixed nuts	168	5	7	15
1 oz. pecans	201	3	4	21
1 oz. walnuts (English)	185	4	4	18